"Lisa Sarasohn is one of the most authentic individuals I have ever known — she lives what she believes. Her message of 'celebration' infuses her teaching, her writing, and her relationships. *The Woman's Belly Book* is the perfect antidote to the media's mission to keep us all buffed, botoxed, and brainless. This book is a terrific resource."

— Adrienne Ressler, MA, LMSW,
national training director of the Renfrew Center Foundation

"This warm and friendly book is filled with womb wisdom, belly laughs, gut feelings, and pelvic power. It is a guide to buried treasure. I recommend it highly."

— Susun S. Weed, author of
New Menopausal Years the Wise Woman Way

"Here is a chance to fill your belly with a banquet of delicious, wholesome advice and inspiration for empowerment and self-esteem. Enjoy!"

— Donna Henes, author of
The Queen of My Self: Stepping into Sovereignty in Midlife

"We desperately need new insights and tools to begin to appreciate, honor, and nourish our core essence and physical being. Many other books inspire us to 'talk the talk' of making peace with our bodies, but *The Woman's Belly Book* shows us how to 'walk the walk.' "

— Margo Maine, PhD, author of
The Body Myth: Adult Women and the Pressure to Be Perfect

"A lovely, wise, and illuminating book that helps women celebrate our bodies and our vital centers. A much-needed antidote to advertising that often makes women anxious about our bodies."

—Jean Kilbourne, EdD, author of
Can't Buy My Love: How Advertising Changes the Way We Think and Feel

"*The Woman's Belly Book* is for every woman who has ever stood in front of her mirror, sucking in her belly, wishing to be different. Lisa teaches us how to cherish the power center within us with a wealth of exercises, modern science, and wisdom from ancient cultures."

— Lavinia Plonka, author of
What Are You Afraid Of? A Body/Mind Guide to Courageous Living

"*The Woman's Belly Book* stimulated a powerful spiritual awakening in me. I became more aware of the spiritual energy available to me. I learned to relax and enjoy my body rather than feeling restricted by it. Viewing my body and my sexuality as sacred greatly enhanced my visceral connection with the source of universal love. Lisa's exercises and words are powerful medicine, graceful and inspiring."

— Elizabeth Fisher, author of
Rise Up and Call Her Name: A Woman-Honoring Journey into Global Earth-Based Spiritualities

"*The Woman's Belly Book* is a blazing trail home to a woman's power, self-esteem, creativity, sexual energy, self-love, and respect for her own beauty. Brilliantly, Lisa opens the veil to women's mysteries, to a place that every woman possesses but hardly dares to venture. Lisa will show you how to honor yourself here and be gentle with what surfaces. *The Woman's Belly Book* is a treasure map to finding and honoring the wisdom deep in you. Let's go mining for truth down there! Are you ready?"

— ALisa Starkweather, founder of the Women's Belly & Womb Conference

"As a researcher and clinician who has spent years trying to help 'solve' women's weight concerns, it's clear to me that it's not another diet or exercise plan that's going to save us. But check out Lisa Sarasohn's winning prescription, helpful for women of all sizes and shapes: drop the negative judgment and celebrate your belly. Finally, a solution — and one that also honors the earth and our community!"

— Linda Bacon, PhD, nutrition researcher, University of California, Davis

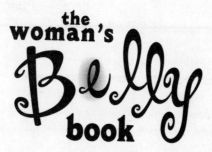

the
woman's
Belly
book

the woman's

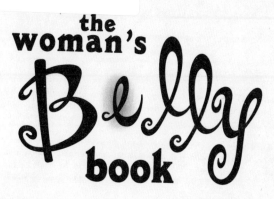

Belly

book

finding your true center
for more energy, confidence,
and pleasure

LISA SARASOHN

NEW WORLD LIBRARY
NOVATO, CALIFORNIA

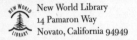 New World Library
14 Pamaron Way
Novato, California 94949

Illustrations by Lisa Sarasohn
Text design and typography by Tona Pearce Myers

Library of Congress Cataloging-in-Publication Data
Sarasohn, Lisa.
The woman's belly book : finding your true center for more energy, confidence, and pleasure / Lisa
Sarasohn.— 1st New World Library ed.
    p.   cm.
Includes bibliographical references.
ISBN-13: 978-1-57731-537-7 (pbk. : alk. paper)
ISBN-10: 1-57731-537-5 (pbk. : alk. paper)
1. Women—Health and hygiene. 2. Yoga. I. Title.
RA781.7.S254 2006
613.7'045—dc22   2005036812

ISBN-10: 1-57731-537-5
ISBN-13: 978-1-57731-537-7
First printing, May 2006
Printed in Canada on acid-free, partially recycled paper

 A proud member of the Green Press Initiative

Distributed by Publishers Group West

10   9   8   7   6   5   4   3   2   1

This book is dedicated to you.

Contents

Welcome

I imagine you're wondering, Is this book for me? Will it make a difference in my life?

This book is about knowing your body's center — your belly — as your center of being, the site of your soul power.

The life force focused in your belly activates your physical, emotional, and spiritual vitality. It's the source of your passion and creativity, your courage and confidence, your capacity to love fully. It's the starting point of your intuition, insight, and sense of purpose. The vital energy centered in your belly is your release from stress, your guide to good health. It is the origin of your inner strength. It's your connection to the source of life itself.

You can develop the Source Energy concentrated in your

body's center. You can direct its expression to enhance every dimension of your life. This book is a guide for doing exactly that.

But still, is this book for you? It's for you if any of the following are true for you:

- You've dieted to trim your tummy or you've crunched your abs to make your stomach flat — without getting the results you want. You're fed up. You want to try a different approach.

- You've had enough of feeling bad about your body. You realize your belly will never be board-flat. You're ready to feel good about yourself as a whole.

- You suspect that if only you could make peace with your belly, you could tap into a wealth of creativity, wisdom, and inner guidance.

- You want to take charge of your sexual energy and fully own your pro-creative power.

- You're getting ready to have a child, and you want to address your concerns about giving birth, mothering, and body image even before you get pregnant.

- You've had a hysterectomy or given birth by cesarean section and still feel torn up. You want to feel whole again.

- You're passing through menopause and want to access the core energy that's becoming all the more available to you at this stage of your life.

◉ You already enjoy yoga, qigong, tai chi, martial arts, African dance, or belly dancing, and you want to experience another approach to body-centered movement.

◉ You're looking for an invigorating, power-centering exercise program you can easily do in five to seven minutes.

◉ You're seeking a body-centered path to personal and spiritual empowerment.

◉ You're a health educator, movement instructor, counselor, bodywork therapist, or health care provider working with women who have any of the concerns listed here.

In addition to a wealth of other material, this book presents The Gutsy Women's Workout as a belly-energizing practice for women with all levels of experience — including no experience at all — in movement arts such as yoga, qigong, tai chi, and belly dancing. And even if you're not interested in developing a movement practice at this time, there's plenty here to engage and reward your attention.

This book *may* be for you — in conjunction with appropriate medical or psychotherapeutic guidance — if you've struggled with an eating disorder, experienced abdominal pain or illness, or survived an assault focused on your belly. Please consult with your health care provider to determine whether and how this book can serve you.

This book is for you to enjoy with the other women in your family as a foundation for fostering respect across the generations.

This book is for you and your friends to use as a basis for mutual support as you find ways to value your belly, your body, yourself.

In these times, it takes guts — courage, determination, and daring — to consider honoring your belly and the soul power it contains. And so I welcome you, a gutsy woman, to *The Woman's Belly Book.*

Introduction

The Treasure
Inside You

This book is and isn't about your belly. It's about the life-giving, life-saving, life-affirming power that already dwells within your body's center — within your belly. This magnificent power is the source of everything I imagine you desire in life: good health, high energy, great sex, unflappable confidence, loving relationships, infinite creativity, meaningful work, unfailing intuition, and an unshakable sense of purpose.

The power focused within your body's center is kin to the Power of Being that creates, sustains, and renews the world. It's the power that, through your body, gives birth to children, generating life itself. It is procreative power in a larger sense as well. It is *pro-creative*, the power to promote creation in any dimension you choose, according to your intention.

This pro-creative life force is your connection to Source Energy. It's your soul in action, your soul power. Where do you rendezvous with this power? In your body's center, within your belly. Whatever your belly's shape or size, this soul power is the priceless treasure inside. In essence, it's who you are.

FINDING TREASURE

Imagine you found a bowl. Maybe you unearthed it when you were digging in the garden. Maybe it's something that caught your eye as you skimmed through a yard sale. However it came to you, this bowl is not necessarily a pretty sight. Its lid is stuck on tight — you can't even open it. It may be scarred or tarnished. It certainly isn't fashionable or stylish. What will people say if you put it on display?

You put the bowl away, in a dark corner of a closet. You're relieved to hide it and forget about it.

Years pass. Then comes the day you're ready to move to a new place. You ask a friend to help you pack. Out of the chaos of cartons, your friend comes to you holding something in her hands. It's the bowl you stowed away all those years ago.

Your friend tells you something surprising. Given what she's learned about antiques, and maybe even archeology, she knows that this bowl is very valuable indeed. What's more, there's something inside. When she holds it up to your ear and gives it a gentle shake, you can hear something rattle.

How will you determine the bowl's true value? Are you going to open it and find out what's inside?

Your friend keeps you company as you consider your options. She tells you what she believes the bowl is worth and how to safely open its lid, if that's what you want to do.

Together with this book, I am that friend. This bowl that you may have forgotten, that you may have hidden with some degree of shame, is your belly. Now, holding this book in your hands, you're on the verge of rediscovering the bowl, your belly, and the priceless something — the treasure — inside.

HOW I LEARNED TO LOVE MY BELLY

This book originated with my own need for healing. I've field-tested all the exercises for deepening awareness and the belly-energizing moves you'll find here. I've needed to — they saved my life.

When I was fourteen, my well-meaning mother presented me with a girdle, something to trim my tummy and slim my thighs so I could wear the straight skirts that were fashionable then. An artifact of the early sixties, this item was the gestapo of girdles. It was so stiff that, when I held it between my hands and tried to pull, it wouldn't give an inch. When I packed myself into it, a diamond-shaped reinforcement panel clamped itself over my tummy, and rectangular reinforcement strips patrolled the outside of each thigh.

The three or four times that I wore this contraption, stuffing my curvaceous belly into this prison for wayward flesh, I could barely breathe. I felt like I was suffocating — the thing was killing me. So I hid it in the back of my bottom drawer and never wore it again.

xviii The Woman's *Belly* Book

But the girdle had already delivered an elaborate message: Your comfort doesn't matter, whether you can breathe doesn't matter, whether you can live fully and freely doesn't matter. What's important is that you look good. If your belly is too big, if it doesn't fit in, you have to hide it, crush it. Your belly shouldn't be seen — it's embarrassing, shameful, wrong. You're a misfit by nature: there's just too much of you. You have to hold yourself in; you don't deserve room to breathe. Don't take up too much space. What's important is that you fit into the very narrow definition of what's acceptable. Left to be yourself, unconstricted, unrestrained, you'll stick out, bulge out, be totally inappropriate.

A few years later, when I was seventeen, I appointed the stick-figured fashion model Twiggy as my ideal of womanhood, my Goddess of Thin. I started dieting. I ate nothing but cottage cheese and drank only water for weeks at a time.

At first, dieting gave me a welcome sense of control. I'd finally found a way to assert my will. When I was dieting I could say, "No, this will not go in my mouth." That sense of control came at a cost, though. In order to restrict my intake of food, I had to override the sensations arising in my belly — not only hunger but also anger, fear, grief, desire, pleasure, and joy.

Dieting delivered this message: You don't deserve nourishment. Food is bad, wrong, dangerous. Your appetites are by definition dangerous. Don't notice what's happening in your belly; those sensations are dangerous and should be ignored. Erase sensation. Empty yourself out. If you feel empty and hollow in your belly, you're doing something right.

My body naturally reacted to such deprivation with an un-controllable craving for food. Weeks of dieting alternated with weeks of binge eating. If I ate one cookie, I'd eat the whole bag.

During the years that followed, I tried one kind of diet after another. The scope of my life narrowed to what I could and couldn't eat, my weight, my shape, what size pants I could squeeze into. I was always on edge, always policing myself.

By the time I was twenty-four, I knew I was losing the war I'd been waging against my belly. It was becoming obvious that I would never find lasting happiness either in consuming another bag of cookies or in squeezing myself into size 7 jeans.

Mercifully, I remembered a yoga demonstration I had wit-nessed as a teenager. Not knowing how else to help myself, I began taking classes in Kripalu yoga — *kripalu* meaning "com-passion" in Sanskrit, the traditional language of yoga. Practicing yoga nurtured my body, eased my mind, and attended to my spirit in ways that food couldn't. I began to live beyond obsession with my weight and shape.

Falling in love with yoga, I trained as a yoga instructor in 1979 and later as a yoga therapist. As part of my continuing training, I learned movement and breathing exercises derived from a Japan-ese style of yoga developed by Masahiro Oki. This approach to yoga focuses on developing *hara* — the Japanese word for the belly as the body's physical and spiritual center, the source of our spiritual power.

The belly as the source of our spiritual power? Who knew? Here was a totally new take on the belly.

As I continued to practice yoga, my eating behavior evened

out quite a bit. I'd still go through periods of bingeing, though, when my emotions threatened to overwhelm me. My eating was nowhere near as frantic as it had been in the past, but there were still times when I felt hopeless. Would this pattern ever change?

One night I woke up from a sound sleep when, apparently, someone turned the light on in my room. Brilliant light filled the space — but, as I quickly learned, my bedside lamp was off.

I don't ordinarily receive visits from the supernatural. In fact, although I keep an open mind, I'm relatively skeptical about paranormal happenings. But I knew that I was dealing with something here, and that I had better sit up and pay attention. I heard a message; a transmission came to me from this blazing light, not so much in words but as knowledge directly conveyed. The message was "Clean up your act with food, or you're going to die."

I noted this instruction, lay back down, and returned to sleep. In the days that followed, I didn't dismiss the message I'd received — it would have been hard to ignore such a wake-up call. But I didn't know what to do with it. I can't say my behavior changed in any way.

About two weeks later, again a bright, blazing light woke me from a sound sleep. Sitting up, I listened for a message. I didn't hear words this time. Instead, I sensed a gesture — the kind of gesture a person makes when she's standing in front of you with her arms crossed over her chest, weight on one foot, tapping the toes of the other foot against the floor. The kind of gesture that says, "Well, we're waiting. We haven't forgotten you. We're watching to see whether you'll ante up." I understood that they (whoever they were) were waiting to see whether I'd do something with myself, rise to the challenge, take charge.

Again, I took this event at face value, lay back down, and returned to sleep.

Not long afterward, I picked up a book I'd been avoiding for a while, Susan Kano's *Making Peace with Food*. The author herself had struggled with the self-starving eating disorder called anorexia. Without mincing words, she pointed out the futile self-absorption of my situation. I heard her saying to me, "How much time and attention are you devoting to worrying about your weight and shape? Why don't you devote that energy and attention to your life purpose instead?"

My life purpose? My life has a *purpose*? Until that moment I hadn't considered that my life had a purpose other than to avoid punishment and please the authorities in their external and internalized forms — my parents, my older sister, my employer, my supervisors. The notion that I had a life purpose was so exhilarating that I didn't care whether I ever found my purpose. It was enough to know that, by birthright, I had one.

Within days, though, a purpose did reveal itself — bright, shining, and clear: I resolved to practice the *hara*-strengthening exercises I was learning on a regular basis. With regular practice, I began to experience the benefits of developing *hara* that I craved — such as more confidence, creativity, and energy and a deeper sense of connection. (See chapter 4 for more on the concept and experience of *hara*.)

After a few weeks of the practice, though, I started feeling a certain nameless dread. So I stopped for a few weeks. Then I took the practice up again for a few weeks. I continued like this, starting the practice and then stopping again. I was running up to the edge of the ocean, sticking a toe in, getting scared, running back to dry land. What was wrong with me?

Energizing my belly was stirring up more than nameless dread, though. One morning, in a room full of seasoned and sober yoga practitioners who, like me, were engaging in this *hara*-strengthening practice, I began to giggle. And I giggled and laughed for half an hour or more, for no reason at all. I began to suspect that whatever feelings were lurking in my belly, they might not all be dreadful. Those feelings hidden deep down in my belly might also include joy.

In 1988, I fully committed myself to the study and practice of *hara*. I made it my purpose to plunge — full-body, full-being — right into the ocean I had been skirting. In the context of this intention, my previous stop-and-start pattern of practicing the belly-energizing exercises was no longer a personal failing. Instead, it became something interesting to investigate. And the nameless dread became nothing more than a clue that something significant was going on under the surface.

I also set my intention to make practical information on developing *hara*, a relatively obscure subject, available in contemporary terms. I resolved to share the good news about our bellies' splendid treasure with a wide audience of women.

And here we are.

Over the years, I've developed a *hara*-strengthening practice that draws not only on yoga but also on movement traditions such as qigong and tai chi. The sequence of twenty-three belly-energizing exercises begins with warm-up stretches that prepare the body for the vigorous moves that follow. The sequence concludes with other stretches for focusing and balancing body and mind. I've been teaching this practice for more than fifteen years, sharing the related insights and skills with hundreds, if not thousands, of women.

Practicing this sequence, along with the exercises for deepening awareness presented throughout this book, I entered into a whole new experience of my body's center. I no longer felt compelled to stuff or starve myself. The eating disorder gradually diminished and disappeared.

Although the initial version of this practice included twenty-three moves, I've created a short form for your convenience in using this book. I've selected seven moves from the original practice and present them here as The Gutsy Women's Workout. Even with this abbreviated sequence — you can easily practice it in five to seven minutes — you'll be reaping the benefits of honoring and energizing your belly.

During my decades of bingeing and dieting, I gained and lost twenty pounds several times each year — at least two thousand pounds in total. I'm sure this repeated weight gain and loss took a physical toll. But even more destructive, my obsession with banishing my belly was dissipating my spirit and unraveling my soul. Discovering my belly as the site of my soul power, my connection to Source Energy, essentially saved my life.

Sharing this process of discovery with you is my greatest joy.

HOW THIS BOOK IS ORGANIZED

This book enables you to cultivate the deep wisdom and creative power concentrated in your body's core.

What's the plan? First, you'll learn five core principles and practices central to reclaiming your pro-creative power. Next, you'll identify the cultural misconceptions that shame women's bellies, preparing you to revalue your belly on your own terms.

You'll also discover that Western culture originally revered the pro-creative power centered in a woman's belly. If in this twenty-first century we choose to honor rather than shame our bellies, we're actually reviving a respectable tradition.

You'll then meet and greet your belly in terms of the many ways it serves you. Taking a tour of the interior, you'll get an insider's view of your belly's physical, emotional, and energetic landscape. You may well discover that your belly is your best friend for your health and happiness in every dimension — that it's literally central to your well-being.

The pro-creative power concentrated in your belly is your soul power, shining through your life as the qualities of vitality, pleasure, confidence, compassion, creativity, intuition, and sense of purpose. Attending to these seven soul qualities in turn, you'll learn specific ways to enhance each one in your life — with opportunities for reflection, journal writing, and art making as well as with belly-energizing breathing and movement exercises. (If you're familiar with yoga, you'll recognize that these seven qualities correspond to the capacities developed through the seven major chakras — spinning wheels of vital energy aligned along your body's vertical axis.)

You'll also find images of seven aspects of your pro-creative power — your powers of cycling, holding space, nourishing, regenerating, expressing, connecting, and being present.

Chapter 13 provides a guide for designing your own belly-energizing practice and incorporating The Gutsy Women's Workout into your life. In this way, the workout becomes a comprehensive exercise in self-respect that empowers you in body, mind, and spirit.

How does our belly-centered soul power relate to the world at large? I'll invite you to consider that humankind's success in surviving on this planet depends on the wise application of our pro-creative power.

Throughout these pages you'll find women's words about their own experiences, reports on the process of becoming belly-proud. These words come from women who have participated in my workshops or who have written to me in response to magazine articles or postings on my website. Consider their voices to be your personal chorus of support.

HOW TO USE THIS BOOK

I suggest you start this book by reading through chapter 1 and becoming familiar with the five core practices: Giving Yourself Room to Breathe, Locating Your Center, Centering the Breath, Naming Your Feelings, and Setting Your Intention. These practices will serve you well as you work with the material in the rest of the book. Having them under your belt, so to speak, equips you to get the most out of the text that follows. Bookmark the pages so you can come back and refer to them at your convenience.

That done, let your intuition — your body knowledge — lead the way. You might, for example, first want to skim the book all the way to the end and get a quick overview, and then start again at the beginning and proceed through the chapters as they're ordered. Or you might want to jump right to chapter 5 and start learning the belly-energizing moves.

I'll say this now and repeat it in chapter 5: As with any other exercise program, before embarking on The Gutsy Women's Workout, check with your health care provider to ensure that the belly-energizing exercises are appropriate for you. Ask your health care provider (and also a seasoned movement instructor) to help you adapt the moves as necessary to accommodate your particular conditions and capacities.

If you're pregnant, be sure to discuss the suitability of The Gutsy Women's Workout for you with your health care provider and childbirth educator. Several of the exercises and some of the breathing patterns include contracting the abdomen. Depending on the stage of your pregnancy, you might want to save the workout for the time after childbirth. But you can still make good use of the Perineal Squeeze in chapter 3 and the gentle breathing patterns offered throughout the book.

If you're not interested in developing a movement practice at this point, that's fine. You might browse through the cultural exposé in chapter 2 and take the belly tour as you read chapter 3. Then you may find yourself curious about some of the breathing patterns in part 2. Several of the exercises for deepening awareness in that part of the book may appeal to you as well.

I've sequenced the awareness and breathing exercises and the belly-energizing movement patterns in order of increasing complexity. If you do pick and choose among them, be sure to observe the guidelines that will enhance your comfort and pleasure as you experiment with them.

Be aware that the awareness exercises — playful ways to begin loving your belly — can also be provocative. They aren't substitutes for professional medical or psychotherapeutic attention. If you become emotionally or physically distressed while doing any of these activities, stop and consult with your health care provider to address your individual needs.

WHAT'S IN THIS FOR YOU?

This book is your invitation to reshape the way you think about, experience, and value your body, your belly, and yourself. You'll discover practical skills for developing the pro-creative power you shelter within your body's center. You'll learn how to direct this power as you choose — for your personal healing as well as for the well-being of your family, your community, and the world.

At this very moment, you're part of a globally expanding circle of women who share this belly-celebrating adventure with you.

Part One

Befriending Your Belly

Chapter One

Core Principles,
Core Practices

This chapter equips you with five fundamental skills, or core practices, for reclaiming your pro-creative power:

- Giving Yourself Room to Breathe
- Locating Your Center
- Centering the Breath
- Naming Your Feelings
- Setting Your Intention

These five core practices enable you to begin honoring your belly in style. You'll encounter these practices in relation to five core principles, which will also guide you on this adventure.

Because this and many other sections of the book invite you to jot down your thoughts and make some drawings, I suggest you supply yourself with a pen or pencil, some colored markers, and some lined and unlined paper. (See Gather Your Supplies on page 8). For writing, I favor inexpensive notebooks; then I don't worry about being messy or making mistakes. You'll want to have at least a pen and some paper handy for the exercises that are coming up.

NOT A SELF-IMPROVEMENT PROGRAM

Here's one of my favorite sentences: This book is not and does not propose a self-improvement program.

Can we say this together?

This is not a self-improvement program.

Thank you.

How do you feel when you say or hear these words? Do you notice a tinge of disappointment? A shred of discomfort as something unfamiliar rises above the horizon? Do you hear a slight tearing sound as these words make a small rip in the idea that there's something wrong with you?

Underneath what may be a tad of disappointment or discomfort, you may notice other feelings. Maybe, at a deeper level, you feel relief, a release of tension. Maybe your shoulders relax and drop down an inch away from your ears. You don't have to defend yourself against charges of wrongdoing. You don't have to protect yourself from attack.

This book is not a self-improvement program. It's not about trying to shove yourself from some grimy Point A, where you are now, to a glittering Point B, over there where you'll be perfect. (We might ask, "Perfect" to whom and for what?)

This book is about discovering, affirming, and being true to who you already are. It's about coming home to yourself and developing the skills to return, again and again, to your center.

I say "again and again" because, after all, what's your purpose here? To finally reach some frozen state of perfection and paste yourself there, unmoving, unbreathing, unchanging? Death may work like that, but life doesn't. Life seems to be about enlarging our experience, expanding the scope of our self-awareness. We experiment, we make mistakes, we go overboard, we lose our balance, we leave home and lose our way for a while. We return. We return again and again, to our center. This book provides you with practical ways to do exactly that.

Sure, you may want to change some of the ways you think, feel, eat, breathe, value, choose, or move. That's fine. The point is to make these changes not to make yourself "better" or "different." The point is to make such changes because they enhance and nourish, amplify and magnify, illuminate and celebrate who you already are.

WHAT IS A "GUTSY WOMAN"?

What is your take on what it means to be a "gutsy woman"? Who are the women who inspire you? What are their qualities?

A GUTSY WOMAN

Let's consider this question: Who are your heroes?

On a sheet of paper, label a column "Women" and make a list, naming five to ten women you admire. Then make a second column titled "Qualities." Across from each woman's name, write down the qualities she embodies, how she inspires you.

Who and what did you come up with?

My list includes poets Alice Walker and Glenis Redmond, activists Rosa Parks and Julia Butterfly Hill, and playwright Eve Ensler. Each has overcome adversity, exemplifying wisdom, grace, and an enduring sense of humor in the process. Each has been outspoken, taking a stand for peace, justice, and the dignity of life. Each has embodied courage and an inner strength that doesn't depend on external approval. Their actions and their words inspire me. They make me feel all the more alive, more at home within myself. By my lights, these are gutsy women.

When I ask these same questions of young low-income single mothers preparing to reenter the workforce, the women often name their mothers — and themselves — as their heroes. They point to the strength and endurance that they and their mothers have demonstrated as they've raised their families with love, no matter how few resources or how little support they've had. These are gutsy women indeed.

Take a look at the list of women you admire and the qualities they embody. I'm guessing the qualities you've named can all be included in the circle of a single word: gutsy. What do you say?

Gutsy: brave, daring, courageous. Self-determined, purposeful. Steadfast, persistent. Sensual, earthy. Creative, compassionate. As the word itself implies, these gutsy qualities don't live in our heads. They're not mental constructs. As Clarissa Pinkola Estés writes in *Women Who Run With the Wolves*, a woman's instinctual knowing "resides in the guts, not in the head."[1] A gutsy woman is a woman who takes charge of the pro-creative power dwelling within her body's center, her belly. Let's play with this some more.

A DAY IN THE LIFE

Write a journal entry describing a day in the life of a gutsy woman. How does she walk, sit, breathe, move, dress, cook, eat, work, deal with conflict, relate to family, speak with friends, make love, sleep? As you write, you might think of the heroes you've named, or fictional characters, or yourself. Let your imagination run free. Whatever you write, you'll be describing aspects of who you already are.

A woman in one of my workshops wrote a poem as part of this exercise, including these lines:

She proudly struts her roundness
The soft comfort speaks of all her strength

GATHER SUPPLIES

If you're getting ready to try out a new recipe, you gather your ingredients. If you're getting ready to travel to a new locale, you gather your gear. This book is an invitation to action. It's a recipe for adventure. Now is the time to gather your supplies.

Here's what you'll need:

Pens or pencils: your favorite writing instruments. Select pens and pencils that allow you to write fast, keeping up with the pace of your thoughts, feelings, sensations, and insights. Keep a few of them handy.

Colors: a set of colored markers with medium tips, or oil pastels. Choose whatever lets you spill lush, bold, vibrant colors onto paper with quick strokes for spontaneity, generosity, and fun. Here's one place to splurge — get the selection of colors that delights you.

Paper: for writing and for doodling and drawing. If you're using individual sheets of paper rather than a notebook or newsprint pad, keep your pages together in a folder or envelope. Choose materials that welcome, even ask for, your wild and spontaneous scribblings. If you're using a notebook, have fun decorating its cover with woman-affirming, belly-honoring images. Always write the date on what you've written or drawn, and title your drawings as you wish.

A container: a box, tote bag, or basket to keep your supplies together with this book and whatever projects may be taking shape. In effect, you'll be creating your own belly-celebrating kit.

Elastic: as in the waistband of the skirt or pants you're wearing as you do the various kinds of exercises. (There's an informal dress code for reading this book and putting it into practice: wear whatever gives your body room to breathe. This code applies to your undergarments, too, of course.)

If you'd like a reason to get yourself a new outfit, here it is. If you were going hiking, you'd want sturdy boots. If you were about to cook up a storm, you'd want an apron. A new outfit is a great way to launch a new adventure in your life. Just be sure that however stylish your new togs might be, they allow you to breathe — fully and deeply.

CORE PRINCIPLE

The best changes occur in our lives when we're nourishing and celebrating who we already are, when we're giving ourselves room to be and opportunities to flourish.

Without judging yourself one way or the other, just notice this: How are you breathing right now? Let's enter into our first core practice, which is all about breathing.

CORE PRACTICE

Giving Yourself Room to Breathe

Are your clothes stifling your breathing? If so, loosen your belt, unzip your zipper, let out your waistband. Take off the tummy-crushing panty hose, shed the tight skirt. Put on something that fits comfortably around your waist and hips.

You can do it. As one woman says, "I don't want to wear anything that interferes with my breathing. Bring on the elastic waistbands!" You deserve clothes that kindly give you room to breathe. Your physical health and your emotional well-being depend on your capacity to breathe deeply. And breathing deeply depends on letting your belly move out and in with each cycle of the breath.

When your belly is free to expand with your inhalation, you can enjoy the benefits of breathing fully, being fully alive.

GIVING YOURSELF ROOM TO BREATHE

1. Sit with your palms resting lightly on your lower abdomen. That's all there is to it. Simply notice the following:

◉ What happens as you breathe?

◉ Which parts of your body, if any, move as you're breathing in and out?

◉ What are your shoulders doing? Your ribs, your waist, your abdomen?

- What's the pace of your breath? Its depth?

- What, if anything, restricts your breathing?

- You may not notice anything. That's fine. Or you may feel your belly moving out and away from your spine with your incoming breath. You may sense it sinking back toward your spine with your outgoing breath.

2. Take a few moments to experience the rhythm of your breathing and how that rhythm plays out in the center of your body. Jot down notes about the sensations, feelings, or thoughts accompanying your experience.

Giving yourself room to breathe is a matter of the highest priority, important enough to be mentioned at auspicious occasions and significant rites of passage. As author Anne Lamott advised graduates during her commencement speech at the Berkeley campus of the University of California in May 2003, "Refuse to wear uncomfortable pants, even if they make you look really thin. Promise me you'll never wear pants that bind or tug or hurt, pants that have an opinion about how much you've just eaten. The pants may be lying!"[2]

You'll find more information on the benefits of breathing deeply in chapter 3, plus a whole array of designer breathing patterns in part 2. The way you breathe reflects and determines your well-being in body and mind. By breathing deeply, you kindle your belly-centered life energy, your power to promote creation.

> After reading about honoring my belly, I bought myself size 24 jeans even though I'm a 20, *just to feel comfy!!*
>
> — *Iona*

THE BODY'S CENTER

Exactly where is the body's center, and why is it so pivotal? The body's center is of prime importance because what happens to the center happens to the whole.

Imagine that you and a friend are ice-skating. Your friend is facing you, standing still. You want to push her across the ice. What do you do?

If you reach out your arm and push on one of her shoulders, she'll turn but she won't cover any distance. But if you put a hand on each of her hips and push on the center of her body, her whole body will move at once, as one, and she will remain in balance. That's the way the world works: what you do to the center you do to the whole.

Your body's center is a point within your belly, a few inches below your navel and a few inches below the skin's surface, a place just in front of your spine. In the realm of physical science, this one point is your center of mass. When your belly center leads you into action, your whole body moves easily, gracefully, almost effortlessly. The whole of you moves as one.

Your body's center is also your center of gravity, the one point that relates all of you to the center of the Earth itself. What happens after you jump into the air? You seem to fall back to the Earth's surface — and you do. The Earth also rises a teeny, tiny bit to meet you.

> I always run with my belly leading when I'm running uphill. It proves to me that the point of center, the point of power, is the belly. And when I come from that place, everything is easier and I can perform better, in any aspect of my life.
>
> — *Tricia*

That's the gravitational bond between your belly center and the Earth's center.

But your belly isn't just your center of gravity. With its abundant supply of iron-rich blood, it is also the center of your electromagnetic field.

YOUR INTUITIVE CENTER: THE ELECTROMAGNETIC FIELD

We gather information about our world, we become aware of ourselves and our environment, through our five senses. I suspect that our awareness also develops through the electromagnetic field infusing and surrounding our bodies.

Our interactions with each other and the world register as changes in our electromagnetic field. Those changes inform what we call our intuition, a perception beyond what we can attribute to our five senses.

The center of a field represents the field as a whole. Where is the center of our electromagnetic field, our intuitive center? Where does our intuition register? In our body's center, in our bellies.

Women and men around the world and throughout time have energized the body's center through dance, healing rites, movement arts, and spiritual practice as a way to cultivate Source

Energy. To name the body's center point and focus on its special significance, they have used phrases that translate, for example, from Korean as "Energy Garden," from Sanskrit as "Luminous Pearl," from Hopi as "Throne of the Creator," and from Chinese as "Sea of Vitality" and "Gate of the Mysterious Female."[3]

In Western culture, references to "the pearl of great price," "the treasure hidden in a field," and even "the fountain of youth" may reveal our longing to rediscover the connection we make with Source Energy through our body's center.

Your body's center — this one point — is the address for your entire self. As Reverend Jeanette Stokes, director of the Resource Center for Women in Ministry in the South, likes to say, it's the "zip code of the soul."[4]

CORE PRINCIPLE

We connect with Source Energy — our soul power, our power to promote creation — through our body's center.

CORE PRACTICE

Locating Your Center

Place your palms on your belly, with the tips of your thumbs touching at your navel and the tips of your index fingers touching below. Notice the triangle that your hands are framing.

Press gently yet firmly into the center of this triangle. What do

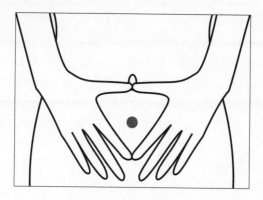

you feel? Your body's center nestles here, deep within the volume of your belly.

Here's another way to locate your center:

LOCATING YOUR CENTER

1. Sit or stand comfortably. Place one palm on your belly, with your thumb at your navel. Place your other palm on your lower back, directly opposite.

2. Let your breathing deepen. As you breathe, imagine a string running from the center of one palm through your body to the center of the other palm. See the string, feel it, describe it to yourself.

3. Find the string's midpoint. Focus your attention at this point for several breaths. What do you observe? Notice the images and sensations that are occurring.

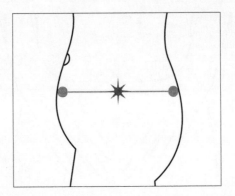

4. Now change the position of your hands and place your palms on your right and left hips, with your thumbs at the level of the bony knobs at the front of your pelvis.

5. Continue breathing deeply. Now imagine another string running from the center of one palm through your body, in front of your spine, to the center of the other palm. See the string, feel it, describe it to yourself.

6. Find and feel where this string intersects the first. Focus your attention at this point for several breaths. What do you observe? Notice the images and sensations that are occurring.

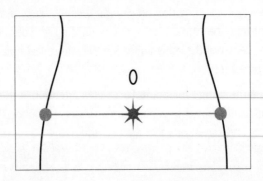

7. Gradually return your attention to your whole body and to the present moment. Write down something about your experience or use color, line, and shape to record the images that emerged and the sensations you experienced.

When you're upset, off-balance, or out of sorts, take a moment to locate your center and put yourself here. Come sit in this garden. When you have "butterflies in your stomach," beckon them to rest on the gorgeous flower that's right here, at your center point.

What other images portray the process of centering yourself? What did you hear as a child? One woman told me, "When I was upset, my grandmother would say, 'Go down and sit in the lap of your angel.'"

How do you name this pivotal point within your belly? Whatever you call it, remember that what happens to the center happens to the whole. Love your belly, and you're on the fast track to loving your whole self.

DO YOU HAVE TO LOVE YOUR BELLY?

Love your belly? Is that really necessary?

As I've said, this book is and isn't about bellies. It's about developing and directing the power to promote creation that's concentrated in your body's center — which, as it happens, is within your belly.

To tap into this power, you have to be willing to deepen your awareness into your belly. You have to let yourself be there, live

there. You have to be willing to let numbness gradually give way
to sensation, to allow blankness and silence to make way for whatever images and messages may want to emerge. You have to let
your belly come alive.

For many, if not most, of us, this is a tall order. For respectable
reasons, many of us have abandoned our bellies; we rarely visit or
call. In chapter 2, I point to the cultural forces that have led us to
make our bellies the objects of our self-hatred. No wonder we've
kept our distance! Working with the exercises in part 2, you'll
have many opportunities to reestablish your mind-belly relationship in a safe and playful way.

"Do I have to love my belly?" I can hear the groan that accompanies the question. You might think that loving your belly is impossible. Right now, I'll settle for your being willing to witness your
judgments about your belly without judging yourself for judging.

CAN I GET A WITNESS?

To enter into and keep returning to witness mode, simply
notice or jot down your judgments about your belly as they
arise. You might repeat them out loud in a high, squeaky
voice or in some other tone that you'd never take seriously.
Don't fight, don't argue, don't resist. Stay neutral, as if you
were simply collecting data on an interesting phenomenon.
Congratulate yourself on the quantity of data you collect —
you're such an attentive observer! — and don't bother yourself about its content.

Do We Have a Deal?

As you become acquainted with your belly from the inside out, you're likely to develop a certain appreciation, even a fondness, for it. As you experience more and more of the vitality, pleasure, creativity, and confidence that energizing your belly brings into your life, you may begin to feel a tad of gratitude. As you reap the benefits of belly awareness in terms of enhancing your relationships, developing your inner guidance, and clarifying your sense of purpose — well, you may find yourself loving your belly after all, no matter what its size or shape. When you're living from the inside out, the view from the outside in becomes irrelevant.

> My daughter Francie met a friend for lunch. The woman confessed, "I shouldn't be eating. I feel so fat; my belly's so big." Francie replied, "If you found something so incredibly precious and powerful that it could bring forth *life*, how would you keep it? Wouldn't you want to wrap it in something soft and round, to cushion and protect it? That something soft and round is your belly."
>
> — *Virginia*

The way I see it, my belly contains the most awesome power imaginable. It's the gateway to my soul, the truth of who I am, the source of every experience I value. If loving my belly is the riddle to solve on the way to uniting with this source, then I'm in.

And you?

Will This Make My Stomach Flat?

This is how it goes: I invite women to consider that our bellies shelter creative energy that's kin to the majestic Power of Being informing the universe. I reveal that it's ours to sample for a bit of compassionate body awareness and belly-energizing movement and breath. And still they may ask me, "Will this make my stomach flat?"

LOVE MY BELLY — ARE YOU KIDDING?

How many times, in how many ways, have you been told that your belly is shameful? How much time and energy have you devoted to banishing your belly, trying to hide it from sight? Is there anything good at all about a woman's belly unless it's flat and hard?

You're right: The idea of loving your belly is challenging. Okay, it's rather unconventional. Given the culture's bias against women's bellies, loving your belly is practically subversive.

But tell me: Whose body is it? Who has the say-so? Who benefits when you belittle your belly? Who benefits when you befriend your belly? What do you get when you give yourself room to breathe?

It's your body, your belly, your life. Whose permission do you need to love yourself?

You're right: Loving your belly is a strange and wild idea. But what's the alternative? Are you willing to abandon the treasure that's so close to home? Or will you do what it takes to claim the treasure that's already yours?

This question packs so much pain inside its six simple words. In chapter 2, I'll invite you to examine the misconception that all women can and should have a flat belly. I'll address the misconception that a round belly makes a woman unfashionable or unattractive.

If you are asking this question, there's another one to consider: What's your underlying concern?

CAN A BIG BELLY BE A SYMPTOM OF SERIOUS ILLNESS?

Abdominal bloating, swelling, or distension can be a sign of disorders affecting digestive and reproductive organs, conditions ranging from food intolerance to uterine fibroids and several kinds of cancer. To eliminate the possibility of a physical ailment, consult with your health care provider — especially if you're experiencing abdominal pain.

If you are at risk for conditions associated with extra fat around your body's midsection, such as diabetes, heart disease, cancer, or stroke, consult with your health care provider to create a plan for minimizing your risk.

In otherwise healthy women, I suspect that extra belly fat can function as protective padding — a shield against self-criticism, a barrier against uncomfortable feelings, or perhaps a buffer against unwanted sexual advances. It's an intriguing possibility: Will replacing self-criticism with self-respect and self-love allow that extra layer of fat to melt away? Engage in the exercises in this book and feel what happens.

Indeed, as you have fun with the breathing and movement patterns outlined in this book, you may notice that you're toning your abdominal muscles. You may witness other pleasing physical changes taking place. Let those changes, when and if they occur, be interesting side effects of coming home to yourself, whatever shape or size your belly may be.

I'm not making any judgments about belly size or shape. I'm not saying small bellies are better than big bellies. I'm not saying round bellies are better than flat bellies. I'm not in the business of judging or diagnosing. I am inviting you to enliven your belly as the source of your inner strength.

In *The Good Body*, Eve Ensler records her quest to make peace with her "imperfect" belly. Her starting point: realizing she had "bought into the idea that if my stomach were flat, then I would be good, and I would be safe. I would be protected. I would be accepted, admired, important, and loved."[5]

Let's take this opportunity to consider how you would feel if your stomach were flat.

IF MY STOMACH WERE FLAT...

Take pen or pencil in hand and complete the following sentences with your own lists:

- If my stomach were flat, then I would have...
- If my stomach were flat, then I would do...
- If my stomach were flat, then I would be...

What do you notice and feel, reading these statements? What are their implications? What other statements and insights follow?

Revisiting the mentality that ruled my life in my twenties, for example, I might write:

◉   If my stomach were flat, then I would fit into my size 7 jeans.

Exploring the implications of this statement, an image might arise:

◉   . . . then I could leave the shadows and jump onstage where everything is well lit and people are dancing and they'd ask me to join them.

And several insights might follow:

◉   . . . then I'd be eligible to be accepted, included, valued.

◉   . . . then I'd be a gen-u-ine human being.

◉   . . . then I'd be real.

Reviewing what I've written, I notice that I'm giving a lot of magical power to these jeans.

Some of your statements might deserve verification. For example, suppose I wrote "If my stomach were flat, then I would be attractive to Terry."

In the spirit of wild adventure, I might then pose the question to Terry in person: "Terry, tell me: if my stomach were flat, would I be attractive to you?"

I might hear Terry reply, "You're already attractive to me. What's the shape of your stomach got to do with it?"

Or Terry might say, "I'm attracted to women who are already confident in themselves and their bodies. If you're not happy with the shape of your stomach, why should I be?"

Or, in a candid mood, Terry might say, "I'm only attracted to women who have flat stomachs. I like to be seen with them because then I feel more powerful myself."

Depending on the answer, of course, you might consider whether Terry is attractive to you.

Now, for the sake of wild experimentation, in the spirit of outrageous play, write these phrases:

- Being who I am, I already have . . .

- Being who I am, I already do . . .

- Being who I am, I already am . . .

Now complete these sentences with exactly the same words you listed in response to the three parallel questions at the beginning of this exercise.

As odd as these new statements might seem, examine them closely for the ways — obvious or subtle — in which they're already true or easily could be true.

Taking the example of the size 7 jeans, my initial statement distilled to "If my stomach were flat, then I'd be real."

Now it becomes "Being who I am, I already am real." Now, that's a rich proposition to consider.

Another example: Suppose I wrote in the first part of the exercise, "If my stomach were flat, then I'd be dating Terry."

Digging deeper for the implications, I continue to discover "...and then I'd have sex...and then I'd have ecstatic experiences in my body."

Moving right along to the second part, I test the possibility "Being who I am, I already have ecstatic experiences in my body."

You may be asking, Is that true? Could that be true for me? I reply, Learn the belly-energizing moves in part 2 of this book, create a delightful and fairly regular practice, and find out for yourself!

CORE PRINCIPLE

Breathing deeply, allowing the belly to move with the breath, activates our pro-creative power and builds our well-being in body and mind.

Are you ready for a breather? The third core practice will literally inspire you as you read and use this book — and as you live your life.

CORE PRACTICE

Centering the Breath

Your first and last breaths are the events that bracket your life on this planet. As long as you're alive here, you'll be breathing. If you're going to be breathing anyway, you might as well give yourself the choice to breathe in a way that adds to rather than drains your vitality; a way that allows you to be relatively relaxed and at the same time alert and attentive; a way that returns you again and again to your center.

You'll find more specifics about breathing and its benefits (in case you need more convincing) in chapter 3. For now, here's one of my stories about the breath.

Years ago the woman who was my supervisor came over to my desk to review a memo I'd drafted. She took a seat in the chair next to me and held the paper in her two hands. As she read, I watched the steady, slow rhythm of her belly expanding as she inhaled, receding as she exhaled. (My breath is deepening right now as I write these words recalling the scene.) I forget what she did or didn't say about the memo. What I'll always remember is the full, deep way she was breathing and the calm, generous, confident presence that seemed to start with her and spread to envelop us both.

DANCE OF THE BREATH

A woman arrived early to pick up her four-year-old daughter, Sara, from dance class. She stood in the doorway and watched as the teacher directed the students to develop their own gestures and move freely to the music. The girls filled the space with their turns and their leaps.

All except one. Sara sat herself down in a corner and watched her belly moving out and in with her breath.

BREATHING AND FEELING

Have you noticed that the way you breathe affects — and is affected by — the way you feel? Remember a time when you were feeling stressed. Recall how you were breathing. Were your breaths deep or shallow? Fast or slow? Quick sips or big slurps? What about a time when you were feeling self-assured — how were you breathing then?

As you witness the link between how you breathe and how you feel, you may discover that a distinctive pattern of breathing corresponds to each of your moods — from sadness and grief to fear and anger, right on through to pleasure and joy. Choose your breathing, choose your mood. We've got designer jeans, designer handbags, designer eyeglasses. Now's the time for designer breathing, and you're the stylist.

The Centering Breath is a pattern of breathing fully and deeply from our bellies, similar to the way we naturally breathed as babies. Since those early days, most of us have been scared and schooled out of this refreshing respiration. Still, our bodies retain the memory and the talent. We can retrain ourselves to breathe as we did at the beginning.

Choose your breathing, choose your mood. Here's an opportunity to discover how the Centering Breath affects your own experience of body and mind. (If you have a serious medical condition, consult with your physician to ensure the suitability of even this gentle breathing pattern for you. Abdominal breathing may not be appropriate, for example, if you have hypoglycemia, diabetes, or kidney disease.)

CENTERING BREATH

1. Set the stage for this deep abdominal breathing by giving yourself room to breathe. Adjust your clothes and your posture to allow your belly to move out and in easily with your breath. Unhitch your waistband, loosen your belt, unzip your zipper. Sit or stand comfortably, adjusting your posture to allow your belly to move freely. Place your palms on your lower abdomen.

2. Notice what's happening underneath your hands. You might already sense a wavelike motion, your belly expanding away from your spine as you inhale and then sinking back toward your spine as you exhale.

3. If you don't see or sense any movement, that's okay. You can jump-start the process by actively pulling your belly in toward your spine as you exhale. Then release the contraction and allow your belly to relax. As it expands naturally — you don't need to push it outward — your belly draws the breath in, beginning the inhalation.

4. Continue, keeping your mouth closed and allowing the breath to move evenly in and out through your nose.

5. Feel the gentle rhythm, allowing your belly to expand and draw the breath in, and then to sink back toward your spine and send the breath out. You might imagine that your belly contains a beautiful balloon. With each inhalation, the balloon fills with breath, and your hands ride with your belly away from your spine. With each exhalation, the balloon

empties; your hands ride with your belly back in toward your spine.

6. Continue observing your belly and your breathing for ten or more cycles of breath.

7. Gradually return your attention to your whole body and to the present moment.

What did you notice and feel? What images and sensations entered your awareness?

You can also practice the Centering Breath lying down, with your feet flat on the ground and your knees bent. Support your knees by placing pillows underneath them, or let them flop inward and rest against each other.

Another option is to place a substantial weight over your lower abdomen. A smooth, round river rock is my favorite; a hefty dictionary will do. Carefully and gently place the weight so that its center of gravity is directly over your body's center, about two inches below your navel. Appreciate the sensation of your strength as your belly rises, filled by the breath, carrying the weight away from your spine and up toward the sky. Enjoy the sense of release as your belly yields, the breath emptying, allowing the weight to sink down toward your spine and the earth.

What did you notice? What did you feel? You'll be encountering these questions often as you experiment with the exercises in this book.

Now let's go on to the fourth of the core principles and practices.

CORE PRINCIPLE

As we deepen our compassionate awareness into our bellies, we increase our receptivity to our gut feelings — the images, sensations, and intuitions arising in our body's center.

Your creativity depends on your willingness to gather the impressions, notice the images, and receive the messages emerging from your body's center. Your intuition does, too. Your intuitions are literally your "gut feelings." They give you important, even life-saving, information.

Yet the feelings stirring in your belly may seem vague, even uncomfortable at times. You can put words to those feelings and receive the information they contain by using images to name your belly sensations.

CORE PRACTICE

Naming Your Feelings

Enlivening your belly means bringing more vitality to your body's center, evoking sensation, stimulating awareness. Many, if not most, of us have cut ourselves off from sensing what's happening within our bellies. The longer we've abandoned this world inside us, the more mysterious — even forbidding — it may seem. But developing and directing your pro-creative power means returning to this territory, investing your awareness here, and claiming it as your own. The process doesn't have to be scary. In fact, it can be fun.

NAMING YOUR FEELINGS

Here's a playful way to name what you're feeling:

1. Consider this list of categories: flowers, fruits, colors, animals, weather conditions, landscapes, fabrics, vehicles, sources of heat. Add your own categories to this list.

2. The sentence below contains two blanks. Choose a category from step 1 to fill in the first blank. Then fill in the second blank with a specific example of that category, using whatever picture or word immediately comes to mind.

    The way my belly feels right now, if my belly were a [category] _____, it would be a [specific example] _____.

    For example, if I chose the category "flowers," my sentence might be "The way my belly feels right now, if my belly were a flower, it would be a red-orange tiger lily.

CORE PRINCIPLE

As we set — and apply our gut determination to — our intentions, we participate in creating our world.

Let's proceed to the fifth and final core practice, which prepares you to begin developing and directing your belly's phenomenal power. It's the skill of setting your intention.

CORE PRACTICE

Setting Your Intention

What is intention? It is awareness informed by purpose, inviting possibility to become actuality. As our world becomes ever more mechanized, digitized, and commercialized, we can be tempted to think of ourselves as machines, formulations, and commodities. We can easily forget that a signature feature of being human is our ability to focus and direct our attention.

As Dr. Larry Dossey reports in *Healing Words: The Power of Prayer and the Practice of Medicine*, some scientific studies have documented the tangible effect that focusing and directing our awareness can have — for example, in the form of prayer for others' well-being. Such research affirms that by articulating our intentions, we participate in creating our world.

If you choose not to specify your intentions, you're likely to see the world as a vague collection of random events to which you have to react. You're likely to feel more or less the victim of a haphazard universe.

When you specify your intentions, you're more likely to perceive events as occurring in coherent patterns. You're an active player in your world. Rather than reacting to random events, you're placing yourself at the center of the action that is your life. You're also organizing yourself (and your electromagnetic field, I suspect!) to attract and receive people and events that support your purpose in mutually rewarding ways.

My intention is to inspire and guide you to develop and direct the power to promote creation that dwells within your body's center. This is awesome power. At this point, you may not believe that this splendid Source Energy resides within your belly. Even if you do believe it's there, you may have doubts about your ability to tap into it. That's fine. You'll discover your own truth in the particulars of your own experience.

For now, work with me here. Suppose this Source Energy does dwell within your body's center. Suppose you can tap into it with compassionate awareness, breath, and movement. How do you intend to use it? How do you intend to direct this creative power in the context of your life?

The exercise in chapter 12 called "Picture Your Heart's Desire" outlines a playful way to set your intention with respect to the pro-creative power you'll be kindling with the belly-energizing exercises. That chapter, which includes the Alignment meditation, addresses the topic of purpose in detail.

The first six belly-energizing moves in part 2, along with the exercises for deepening awareness, prepare you to practice the final move, Alignment, with integrity. You'll be ready to witness how practicing the whole power-centering sequence contributes to fulfilling your intentions and making your dreams come true.

Yes, the creative power concentrated within your body's center is an awesome power. Some women tell me that at first, experiencing this energy can be somewhat daunting. As they clarify their intention for using this energy, though, the uneasy feeling gives way to a welcome sense of affirmation.

Setting your intention and picturing your heart's desire will help you feel safe as you learn and practice the belly-energizing moves. Setting your intention right now is important, too. Doing so will help you feel comfortable as you work with this book and continue on the adventure of honoring and enlivening your body's center.

SETTING YOUR INTENTION

What's your pleasure? I love hearing those words. They tell me that there's no limit to how I can define my desire. What's your pleasure? Leave any idea of restriction or limitation behind as you begin setting your intention for the adventure that awaits you.

1. Take a moment to clear your mind. Get comfortable; give yourself room to breathe fully and deeply. Let some of your attention rest within your belly.

2. Consider these questions: What drew you to this book? How do you intend to use it? What benefits are you willing to receive?

3. Let words, phrases, and images emerge into your awareness. When you're ready, take pen or pencil in hand and let your words spill out onto paper. Use colors to doodle the lines, shapes, and forms that come forth from your inner knowing, revealing some aspects of your intention.

4. When you've finished, title and date your drawing. Post it in a place where you can see and enjoy it often.

From time to time, review your intention. Return to this process to keep the image of your intention up to date with what's important to you.

CORE PRINCIPLES

1. The best changes occur in our lives when we're nourishing and celebrating who we already are, when we're giving ourselves room to be and opportunities to flourish.

2. We connect with Source Energy — our soul power, our power to promote creation — through our body's center.

3. Breathing deeply, allowing the belly to move with the breath, activates our pro-creative power and builds our well-being in body and mind.

4. As we deepen our compassionate awareness into our bellies, we increase our receptivity to our gut feelings — the images, sensations, and intuitions arising in our body's center.

5. As we set — and apply our gut determination to — our intentions, we participate in creating our world.

Chapter Two

A Cultural Exposé

Here in the early years of the twenty-first century, exposing the abdomen with high-cut crop tops and low-slung jeans is all the rage. Let's see how the abdomen has fared in our history and culture, looking through the lens of some common misconceptions.

FIVE MISCONCEPTIONS ABOUT WOMEN'S BELLIES

The simple truth: Unless you've escaped the influence of television, movies, books, newspapers, magazines, comics, dress-up dolls, family, church, school, and friends, you've been bombarded with millions of messages shaming your belly. You know how it goes. Magazine covers blare "Lose Your Belly!" and display fashion models whose abdomens have likely been airbrushed out of the picture. Advertising in magazines and on television pushes diet plans and pills. In television programs and films, the thin girls get their man on their way to stardom. (We don't see the faces of the women who stand in as body doubles when even the stars' bellies and butts don't make the grade.)

There are only a handful of supermodels and Hollywood stars. Should the rest of us make ourselves miserable trying to look like them?

The shame that besets us about our bellies can go to extremes. One woman, for example, told me, "Once I was so sick that I had to call an ambulance to take me to the hospital. As the medics were taking off my shirt — I was practically dying — all I could think about was sucking in my belly so they wouldn't see my fat stomach."

Our insecurities about our bellies bankroll the weight-loss, diet products, plastic surgery, advertising, media, shapewear, cosmetics, and fitness industries. Consumed by the idea that there's something wrong with our bellies, we're ready to trade our money for the fixes such industries are pushing. We're primed to purchase one product or service after another.

But the insecurities that make us such steady, compliant consumers are artificially induced; we're not born with them. As Jean Kilbourne documents in *Can't Buy My Love: How Advertising Changes the Way We Think and Feel*, the industries that stand to benefit from our continuing quest to "improve" our bodies carefully and cleverly cultivate our anxieties.

The good news is that we don't have to swallow the misconceptions — call them lies, if you like — that such industries have been broadcasting. We don't have to let some corporate exec send us shopping for what we really don't need.

As you recognize these misconceptions for what they are, you can choose for yourself how to value your body's center. As you disabuse yourself of these deceptions, you can make the choices that truly enhance your health and well-being.

MISCONCEPTION #1

Women of all ages can and should have a flat belly.

Nature does not intend a woman to look like a ten-year-old boy. In fact, nature designs a woman's belly to shelter and nurture new life. A woman's belly holds and protects her womb, promoting the survival of the human species.

Nature expresses itself through genetics. A small percentage of women may have genes that allow for a fat-free midriff — when they're in their teens and twenties. The rest of us have the honor of displaying nature's more curvaceous design.

Our culture tells us that the best belly is the one that you cannot see, the one that's invisible to the eye. This stricture leads us to assume that we can control the shape and size of our bellies if we want to, if only we try hard enough — and if we buy enough of the right products and services. Just what is it we're trying to control, and why?

I've made field trips to the lingerie sections of local department stores. I've leafed through mail order catalogs for sportswear. I've studied the literature attached to girdles and shapewear of all sorts. I've pondered the benefits they promise. The promotions for these undergarments read like an FBI directive for suppressing foreign insurgents: "Achieve firm control . . . obtain total control . . . eliminate undesirable elements." There's the evidence: the girdle is an instrument of social control.

The power we hold within our bellies is the power to promote creation, to bring something new into being. From the point of view of any authority invested in keeping things the way they are, a woman's ability to develop and express this power could seem subversive.

The power we hold within our bellies is revolutionary indeed. More precisely, it's evolutionary. Our body-centered wisdom, our gut knowing, is our instinct for self-preservation. It speaks to our survival as individuals and to the survival of our species. If heeded, such body-centered wisdom can help the tribe of human beings adapt to the emerging actualities of life on this planet. Still, such change, and the wisdom calling for such change, can seem threatening.

A woman's belly is not a machine. It's not a lump of clay. It's not dead weight. It's not made of stuff you can pick up at the hardware or fabric store. As I'll invite you to consider in chapter 4, your belly is a sentient — meaning feeling, knowing, caring, sensing — being. It's alive, just as you are alive. It has its own story, its own trials and triumphs. It stores messages that you've put on hold until you're ready to attend to them. In its size and shape, as well as in the way it functions, your belly embodies the truth that's central to your well-being.

If a woman did all the approved fat-burning aerobic exercises, the ab-attacking routines, and the tummy-trimming diet plans, would she succeed in making her belly flat?

Maybe, maybe not. I suspect that if my belly is protruding, it's trying to bring something to my attention. If I try to flatten it with all the delicacy of pounding on it with a hammer, I'll miss the message it's been holding for me. And whatever information my belly has been trying to insert into my awareness through a bit of bloating or an extra layer of fat will have to find another, probably more uncomfortable, way to catch my attention. When I'm willing to address the core issue my belly has been embodying, the bloating dissipates and the extra layer of fat melts away. (Chapter 4 elaborates on decoding the body's symptoms of distress.)

The shape of a woman's belly may also reflect the shape that our environment is in. Man-made pollutants, pesticides, and agents of disease are increasingly prevalent in our air, water, food, and medicine. We're increasingly exposed to contaminated vaccines, chemicals sprayed into the air for weed control and weather modification, and genetically engineered bioweapons. Such substances present toxins our bodies don't know how to neutralize, exceeding our immune system's capacity to respond.

As we're exposed to these substances, our bodies attempt to protect us however they can. Our bellies, for example, may attempt to contain and cordon off genetically engineered viruses with an overgrowth of candida, the yeast that naturally occurs in the large intestine in moderate amounts. An overgrowth of candida can cause abdominal bloating and other signs of abdominal distress, which ab crunches and weight-loss diets won't necessarily address.

Toxic substances can also interfere with the function of organs involved in fat and carbohydrate metabolism, resulting in weight gain that isn't easy to reverse. Such toxins can also interfere with the action of reproductive hormones and play a part in menstrual pain and menopausal discomfort.

What is your body's relationship to our environment? Your body is the portion of this home planet that you personally inhabit. I suspect that if we wish to savor our body's naturally elegant curves and the natural sleekness of our bellies, we must also act to save the earth's air, water, and soil from destruction.

THE SHAPE OF BEAUTY

During the next few days, be on the lookout for beauty. What do you see, hear, touch, taste, and smell that's beautiful? Is beauty uniform, fixed, straight, angular, flat? Is it textured, variable, smooth, sloping, curved? What makes something beautiful to you?

Our culture prizes the curve of a woman's breast but not the curve of her belly. What do you make of that?

MISCONCEPTION #2

Big-bellied women have always been unfashionable in Western culture.

Although current fashion dictates shrinking a woman's belly from sight, in other times enormous bellies were in vogue. In

Europe, from the fifteenth through the seventeenth centuries, for example, men judged a woman to be as sexually appealing as her belly was large. "In the erotic imagination of Europe," writes Anne Hollander in *Seeing Through Clothes*, "it was apparently impossible until the late seventeenth century for a woman to have too big a belly." Accordingly, women's apparel enhanced the belly's size: "All dress for women was unvarying in its emphasis on the stomach.... A woman's belly provided the central accent point of her costume."[1]

Fashions in women's physical form have come and gone through the centuries. But, as Naomi Wolf points out in *The Beauty Myth*, a turning point occurred in the early twentieth century when women in England and America gained the right to vote. Since that time, the womanly belly has steadily lost favor. As women began to participate in the "man's world" of politics and government, the belly — the literal and figurative sign of womanly power — became, ideally, invisible.[2]

Archeological evidence suggests that we humans originally imagined the Power of Being in womanly form as the Mother of the Universe. In *The Language of the Goddess*, Marija Gimbutas demonstrates that the forebears of European culture produced figurines, engravings, ceramic designs, paintings, and earthworks that acknowledged the power of the Great Mother's ample belly to birth, nurture, and renew the world. The art that our ancestors made, beginning with the outline of vulvas etched into cave walls, honored a woman's belly as the source of life itself. Our ancestors considered a woman's belly to be sacred, not shameful. Maybe our ancestors got it right.

BELLY PICTURE BOOK

Make a picture album that shows how women's bodies and bellies have been portrayed through time and across the globe. Include modern-day magazine advertisements, copies of historical photographs, and representations of women in painting, drawing, and sculpture through the ages. Add pictures of fashion models, celebrities, and religious figures as well as of "ordinary" women. Include photos of women in traditional dress from cultures around the world.

Notice what you feel when you look at these pictures. What do you see about these women and their bellies?

MISCONCEPTION #3

The best thing you can do for your belly is to make your abdominal muscles rock-hard. Hold your breath in and "suck it up" all day.

Your physical, emotional, and spiritual well-being depends on your capacity to breathe fully and deeply. By making your abdominal muscles rigid, you restrict your breath. When you don't give yourself room to breathe, you're reducing your vitality. You're cutting yourself off from life.

As a seasoned bodyworker, I've had the privilege of touching many women's bellies. As my palms rest on a woman's belly, my hands receive information through the texture and temperature of the skin, the muscles' tone, the pulsing of blood, and the resiliency of the tissue in relation to the pattern of breath.

One day I worked with a young woman who, to all appearances, was trim, fit, and fashionably thin. Her belly was fashionably flat as well. When I gently laid one palm on her belly, what I felt was hard, cold, unmoving. Rigid, bitter, adamant refusal. This woman's belly was as hard and flat as a prison wall. It was freezing her out of life, enforcing her isolation, giving her absolutely no room to breathe.

What would you wish for this woman, and for yourself? Which would you prefer: a hard, flat, immobile belly that cuts you off from life, or a nicely rounded, resilient belly that moves with the ebb and flow of the breath?

There's nothing useful about making your belly rock-hard and restricting your breath. Your time on this planet is determined by the number of breaths you take. Your life is as satisfying as the quality — the depth and fullness — of your breathing.

You can tone your abdominal muscles without making them tight. And that's a good thing to do. Strengthening these muscles means they can give all the more support to your spine and help relieve pain in an otherwise overworked lower back. Strengthening these muscles also increases their capacity to support your abdominal organs.

Strong muscles in your midsection stabilize your torso and make a sturdy foundation for the work all your other muscles are doing. Stabilizing your trunk equips you to move with more balance and flexibility; it can increase your endurance and help you avoid injury.

Attacking the abs takes its toll, though. Incorrectly performing Pilates exercises unbalances the body. Overdoing sit-ups and crunches leads to injury. The unpleasant effects include flattening the curve in the lower spine, which weakens the spine as a whole; rounding the middle spine and shoulders into a permanent hunch; and inflaming the discs between the spinal vertebrae, which makes sitting, bending over, and lifting extraordinarily painful.

One woman, for example, worked out intensively at the gym, doing sit-ups plus dozens of reps on the ab machines to flatten her belly. The result? Her back rounded into a prominent and disfiguring dowager's hump.

Another woman reveals that she's been "sucking her belly in" since she was ten. Yes, her belly is flat — and her muscles are habitually tense. What was she trying to accomplish? Her goal, she says, was to be "the supermodel version of 'slim,' meaning ultra-thin, no matter whether it was healthy or not. When I was very, very young, I read a romance novel that mentioned the heroine's flat belly and the fact that she did not need a girdle. I grew up in the days when no self-respecting young girl or woman would dare leave the house without a girdle to squeeze her into shape. My body type is slender. But that poor, tortured, over-exercised belly was never flat enough for me, never. Did I ever see the 'real' me? Never. Only the role assigned by the media: flat belly. I don't even remember what it was like not to pull those abs in tight. I did it in my sleep, even."

What were the results? "A case of such incredibly tight abdominal muscles that they pulled my lumbar spine into permanent flexion [forward bending], flattening out my natural lumbar curve. A state of permanent tension. An absolute inability to feel my own life energy. I was (and still am) completely shut down internally. My belly feels like a rock most of the time."

But there's more: her success in flattening her abs may have contributed to pushing her uterus and bladder out of place. "These strong muscles did not keep my abdominal organs from prolapsing, and I have a very irritating leaky bladder. I have had two major abdominal surgeries, one a hysterectomy at the tender age of twenty-nine due to the severity of my prolapsed uterus, and another because of the adhesions and scar tissue resulting from that hysterectomy."

MISCONCEPTION #4

Girdles, control-top panty hose, and tight pants are harmless.

Girdles not only are instruments of social control — they can be lethal as well. Fortunately, tight-laced corsets are no longer in fashion. In the not-too-distant past, however, many women wore them every day. As a result, their abdominal muscles atrophied, becoming useless.

As one woman remembers, "My mother wore a girdle every waking minute until she was more than eighty years old, when the pain and compression of her abdomen demanded that she stop. By then she had no muscle tone of her own that would have kept her organs in place."

A corset could also compress a woman's belly to the point of causing gastroesophageal reflux disease (acid reflux, or GERD). As the acidic contents of the stomach were forced up and breathed back in, they scarred the lungs and made them vulnerable to infection. Repeated episodes of the aspiration pneumonia that followed led eventually to fatality — death by corset.3

In the early years of the twenty-first century, shapewear is making it to market in a variety of forms. Designers are incorporating girdles into swimsuits, panty hose, skirts, and jeans — jeans priced at nearly $200, that is.

As the next chapter details, anything that constricts your belly and restricts your breathing reduces the amount of oxygen getting to your body and brain, taking away from your physical and emotional vitality as well. But that's not all. The culture's obsession with trimming women's tummies interferes with even more than women's health.

Americans — primarily women, I suspect — spend more than $40 billion on figure-shaping each year. What else could we do with that money? If we bought $10 jeans instead of $200 jeans, what could we do with the $190 we've saved?

How much of our attention do we devote to belittling our bellies, attacking our abs as if they were the enemy? What would our lives be like if we attended instead to developing and directing the creative power concentrated in our bellies according to our conscious intention?

There's a saying that the emperor Nero fiddled while Rome burned. We women may likewise be frittering away our time, money, energy, attention, and creative power as the fabric of life on this planet unravels.

MISCONCEPTION #5

A round belly on a woman means she's lazy, gluttonous, and slutty; her appetites are insatiable.

A woman's belly is a symbol with great significance. It's a robust visual reminder that a woman's body contains an awesome power — the capacity to bring forth new life. It also signifies a woman's capacity to feel and fulfill her desires, to nourish herself by taking in and processing food. A woman's rounded belly is visible evidence of her capacity for both reproduction and digestion — for both construction and destruction, both birth and death.

> My mother made me wear a girdle when I was a teenager, even though I was pencil-thin. "Nothing should shake," she'd say. "Ladies don't shake." I think that if we didn't waste our energy on worrying about our size and shape, we could move the world!
>
> — *Ann*

This balanced capacity to bring forth and to tear apart reminds us that the power to promote creation is balanced as well. It's a continuing process of bringing in the new, sustaining it while it works, wiping it away when it's no longer useful, and preparing the way for the next generation. The uterus itself goes through such a process in the monthly cycle of menstruation.

The unchecked impulse for growth — in our cells, in our lives, in our economies, among our nations — leads to cancer, greed, hunger, and war. Unlimited growth eventually destroys life itself. If life is to continue, the cycle of creation must include endings. The life-affirming power we carry within our bellies includes the capacity to know what's enough, to say "no" and "stop" and put an end to things. It includes the capacity to take things apart and reduce them to their elements, and to reorganize the elements into something new. Our pro-creative power ushers life through the full cycle of birth, growth, death, and renewal.

Archeological artifacts indicate that our ancestors revered women's bellies both as wombs of creation and as tombs of regeneration. Ancient icons show woman as mistress of both birth and death.

A woman's ample belly is a visual reminder of her awesome power to create life, akin to the Power of Being that creates our world. Her belly is evidence of her tangible connection to the source of life that brings forth, sustains, and renews the universe. Her belly also reminds us of the mystery that awaits us beyond our last breath.

FEAR AND LOATHING

The misconceptions about women's bellies reflect Western culture's fear and envy regarding the pro-creative power our bellies shelter. (Can you say "womb envy," Dr. Freud?)

I've heard many women say that their bellies are, or have been, the focus of their self-loathing. The way I see it, such self-loathing is a personal response to a cultural process of invalidation. Our culture has made a habit of devaluing women and demeaning our bellies. The problem is not with our bellies. The problem is with our culture.

There's nothing inherently wrong or bad about a woman's belly. If I agree to be ashamed of my belly, then I'm participating in my own oppression. If I abandon my body's center, I'm giving away my own power.

Although egalitarian, woman-honoring societies continued to

flourish in prehistoric Europe and the Near East for millennia, in the past five thousand years, Western civilization has witnessed the devaluation of women and the appropriation of women's power. Cultural, religious, political, legal, and economic institutions have attempted to control, exploit, and usurp the pro-creative power we women shelter within our bellies. In a single process of desecration, as Western culture has devalued women and shamed our bellies, it has also exploited native peoples, degraded nature, and marginalized emotional sensitivity among men.

Our culture exposes women's bellies to overt and covert violence. It frames women's bellies as targets of assault, resources to exploit, and objects to control.

The study of cultural violence against women and women's bellies can be gut-wrenching. It's also liberating. It shows that whatever shame we might feel with respect to our bellies, the shame wasn't our idea — it's an artifact of culture. The shame is only ours if we choose to make it so.

You'll find some of the gruesome details of the culture's violence against women and our bellies in appendix 1. I don't want to belabor the point here. Look into these details when you're ready.

BELLY CELEBRATION

In contrast to contemporary Western culture, women and men in other times and places have admired women's belly-centered power. Through myth, ritual, image, traditions of dance, and spiritual practice, these people have expressed their reverence for and desire to participate in this power. The role of Baubo in the Greek myth of Demeter and Persephone, the legendary search for the Holy Grail, and the practice of walking the labyrinth demonstrate three of the many ways in which cultures around the globe have celebrated women's bellies and the pro-creative power we shelter in our body's center.

The Belly Goddess

In the myths, rituals, and sacred images of many civilizations, the womanly belly is a goddess. The ancient Greeks named their belly goddess Baubo and gave her the pivotal role to play in Demeter's search for her daughter. Baubo makes the difference between the life and death of the world.

In this story, Hades has raped and abducted Demeter's daughter, Persephone, taking her away to his underworld realm. Demeter — also known as the earth goddess, Gaia — is devastated. The earth reflects her despair; the crops die and the fields become barren. Famine threatens humankind's survival.

Demeter, nearly immobilized by grief, arrives at a place called Eleusis. Baubo comes to stand before her. She tells bawdy jokes, dances a hip-wiggling jig, lifts her skirt, and flashes her vulva. Baubo's rowdy antics make Demeter laugh and laugh. Seeing Baubo bare her belly, Demeter remembers who she is and the power that she holds.

The belly laughter that Baubo provokes dispels Demeter's depression and restores her will. Now Demeter has the guts to continue looking for her daughter. She eventually finds Persephone, and the earth becomes fertile again, saving humankind from extinction.

The ancient Greeks enacted this story annually in the Eleusinian Rites, a secret initiation. The details of the ritual remain a mystery. The reports we do have, however, suggest that those who participated in the ritual lost their fear of death. In some manner, they received a taste of eternal life.

The belly goddess personifies — deifies, really — the power of life to reach beyond death. She is the life-restoring force not only in the Greek story of Demeter but also in the Egyptian myth of Isis and in the Japanese myth of the sun goddess Amaterasu. The belly goddess figures in the stone carvings that ornament English and Irish churches, European cathedrals, and Indian temples. She appears in Eastern European embroidery and in motifs that have appeared for thousands of years in Africa, Asia, the Pacific islands, and the Americas. Such images are kin to the engravings that our earliest ancestors etched into cave walls. The belly goddess, in her many names and guises, lives in the origins of human consciousness. She is the sacredness of women's bellies.

Indeed, the links shown by language suggest that the Greek Baubo is a later, reduced version of the Great Goddess — known in the Middle East as the Sumerian Bau, the Phoenician Baev and Baau, and the Syrian Baalat.[4] In the wholeness of experience, perhaps there is no belly goddess apart from the Great Goddess herself, the Power of Being immanent within our body's center.

The Holy Grail

In some legends, the Holy Grail is the cup from which Jesus drank at the Last Supper. In others, it's the cup into which Joseph of Arimathea collected Jesus's blood as he died on the cross. Possibly, it's a set of documents that prove Mary Magdalene was the wife of Jesus and the mother of their child. Perhaps it's a reliquary containing Mary Magdalene's remains. The Holy Grail — *San Graal* in Old French — might refer to Mary Magdalene herself. The Grail, then, is the emblem of her pregnant belly as she carried Jesus's royal blood — *sang raal* — into another generation.

Whatever the Holy Grail might be in legend or fact, it's often pictured as a stemmed cup, a chalice, signifying the source of life everlasting. The quest for the Grail is the quest for eternal life.

The form of the chalice contains its meaning. The geometric proportions that shape the chalice are the same as those that locate the body's center along the vertical axis of the human body. The basis for these proportions, in both chalice and body, is the square root of 2.

From ancient times to the European Renaissance, artists and architects incorporated the numerical relationships found in nature into their designs. They perceived that the proportions ordering the natural world revealed universal principles. Embedding the same proportions into their constructions, they imbued their work with sacred meaning.

What is the significance of the square root of 2? In the tradition of Sacred Geometry, the square root of 2 (also written as $\sqrt{2}$) represents the transformation of One into Two, the power of doubling. The implicit meaning of $\sqrt{2}$ is generation. The root of 2 is the source, the root, from which life proceeds.[5]

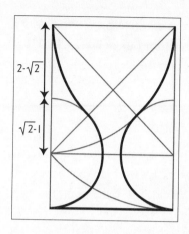

The form of the chalice
incorporates the square root of 2
into its proportions.

Given the geometry of its form, the chalice is a visual code for
the self-generating source of life. At the same time, it's a code
for the life force located in the body's center.

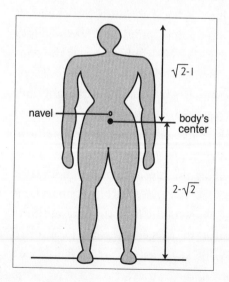

Proportions incorporating
the square root of 2 locate the
body's center along the length
of the human body.

The Holy Grail signifies the pro-creative power that Mary Magdalene and all women shelter within our bellies. The Holy Grail is every woman willing to contain the sacredness of life and carry it forward.

The Labyrinth

The labyrinth defines a path into and out from center. As a sacred symbol, it maps a journey from the everyday world to the secret core of existence. It charts a path to the World Navel, the point through which the life force emerges to revitalize the world.[6]

From ancient times, cultures throughout the world from the Arctic to Africa have made labyrinths in a variety of designs. The labyrinth appears on cave walls, stone slabs, grave markers, pottery, coins, and the bellies of clay figurines. When laid out with pebbles or standing stones on the ground, or embedded into sanctuary floors, the labyrinth serves as the template for sacred dance. Although many associations accompany the design, in some traditions the labyrinth clearly signifies a woman's belly. The path through the pattern traces the soul's return to the womb and its emergence in rebirth.

When my daughter was a toddler, when she met someone for the first time, she'd lift her shirt up and show them her belly.

— Tori

The word *labyrinth* means "house of the *labrys*." The labrys is the double-bladed ax invoking the presence of the goddess. It signifies the power of the goddess to regenerate life. With its convex blades, the ax reveals the shape of the butterfly and recalls its transformation from caterpillar to winged creature. The open crescent of the ax's upper edge suggests the arc of the uterine tubes curving from the uterus to the ovaries.

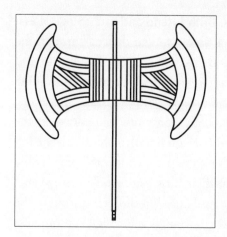

A labrys, a double-bladed
ax. Minoan, Crete,
2nd millennium B.C.E.

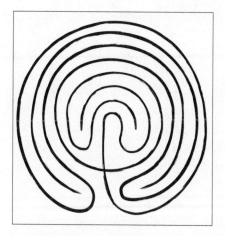

Labyrinth design on a coin.
Knossos, Crete,
1st millennium B.C.E.

The house of the labrys, then, is literally the sanctuary enclosing the icon of a woman's pro-creative power. The labyrinth is the
body of the goddess, enclosing her womb.

The original House of the Labrys is within the Palace of
Knossos on the island of Crete, named for the many signs of the

labrys ornamenting its walls. Both legend and archeological evidence suggest that in ancient times women danced through the labyrinth at the Palace of Knossos, red scarves tied end to end threading through their hands and held at their hips. One woman, Ann-Adele, visited Knossos with a group of friends. They walked in pairs through the labyrinth embedded in the palace's floor. In each pair, one person put on a blindfold; she followed her sighted partner along the path, connected only by the red ribbon they each held at their hips. Ann-Adele learned that to keep her balance while walking blindfolded through the labyrinth, she had to trust her gut feelings, allowing her awareness to sink down from her head to her belly.

WALKING THE LABYRINTH

One Sunday night, the sanctuary of the church I attend was entirely clear except for an enormous sheet of canvas that covered the floor. Drawn on the canvas was an actual-size replica of the labyrinth that's embedded in the stone floor of France's Chartres cathedral, dating to the thirteenth century.

The woman who brought the replica introduced the labyrinth to the hundred of us who had gathered. She told us something about its history and significance, and she invited us to walk it, to enter the design when we felt moved to do so.

As she was speaking, I could barely wait for the chance to begin. My body rocked back and forth, my belly throbbed with insistent yearning. I felt a reaching from the center of my womb as if there were a magnet there being drawn irresistibly to the mother lode at the labyrinth's center. This great hungry need felt ancient in origin, urgent, not to be denied.

Once we were invited to begin, I couldn't wait a moment longer. When I rose and walked to the labyrinth's entrance, my immediate impulse was to kneel and stretch my body out full-length, bringing my belly to the canvas-covered floor. My body crawled forward through the first straight passageway in a passion that pressed my belly to the earth, pulled toward the labyrinth's center.

At the end of that first straight segment, I rose from the ground to walk, then dance, the turns. Each of the labyrinth's curves had its own nature, its own flavor. Reaching the petals at the center, I felt a surge of life energy rushing up through my body, as if I were standing within a fountain of joy. I played in that fountain, tracing the vertical current, sensing the energies converging and interchanging at this central point.

When the time came to return, I didn't want to leave the center. I left reluctantly. The ordinary outside world, I thought, would be dingy compared to those moments of pure bliss I'd experienced at the center.

On my way out of the labyrinth, I learned that the purpose of journeying to the center is not to hide there, not to disappear into the numinous. The journey's purpose is to dip into that shining essence and remember, be refreshed. That refreshment enables me to return to the "ordinary" world and be more present to the grace that already suffuses it.

The labyrinth establishes the center and protects it; the design determines how you approach the center and how you leave it. As you travel, the circuitous route invites you to shed your outer layers, your deceptions, illusions, affectations. Moving through the labyrinth requires courage, faith, and tenacity; at times the path takes you farther away from the center, not closer to it.

Finally arriving at the center, you step into the mystery. How do you experience the grace that awaits you?

The journey outward poses the questions, How will you bring the renewal you've found at the center out into the world? Are you willing to return to the world and see the center anywhere, and everywhere?

VENTRILOQUISM

When you're speaking your gut truth, you're practicing the ancient art of ventriloquism. *Ventriloquism* means, literally, "speaking from your belly," voicing the language of your *venter*. *Venter* is a word of Latin derivation meaning "belly," "womb," and "woman as birth-giver."

In current usage, a ventriloquist is an entertaining trickster, projecting the voice without moving the lips, producing the illusion that someone or something else is talking. Originally, ventriloquism was the practice of priestesses, women speaking from their bellies to deliver oracular wisdom, conveying the voice of the goddess emerging from the earth.

We can trace how the meaning of *ventriloquism* and related

words has changed over time in a sampling of references cited in the *Oxford English Dictionary*:7

The Bible's book of Isaiah makes reference to "a voice which whispers out of the ground like a familiar spirit." Conybeare and Howson, writing in *St. Paul*, claim that "It was usual for the prophetic spirit to make itself known by an internal muttering or ventriloquism."

As women honoring the goddess came to be classified as witches, ventriloquism came to be associated with witchcraft. The voice that emerged from the belly — what was once considered to be oracular wisdom — came to be feared as diabolical. In his 1584 treatise on witchcraft, R. Scot describes a "wench, practising hir diabolicall witchcraft and ventriloquie." In 1644, Digby warned that ventriloquists "do persuade ignorant people that the Diuell [Devil] speaketh from within them deepe in their belly," and in 1656, Blount defined a ventriloquist as "one that hath an evil spirit speaking in his belly."

Similarly, in 1680, Glanvill wrote that "Ventriloquy, or speaking from the bottom of the Belly, 'tis a thing as strange as anything in Witchcraft." He characterized one who speaks from the depths of her belly as a Pythoness. In his usage, *Pythoness* meant "witch" in a derisive sense. But, appropriately, the term originally referred to soothsaying women such as the priestesses of Delphi, who expressed the oracular voice of the underground serpent, the current of primordial life force generating the world. The serpent-priestess also fig-ures in Kingsley's 1855 exhortation to "discourse eloquence from thy central omphalos [navel], like Pythoness ventriloquising."

By the early nineteenth century, ventriloquism had become a

parlor trick and a theatrical entertainment. An 1815 issue of *Stage*, for example, reports that "A ventriloquist at Paris has attracted the attention of the whole metropolis." Speaking from the belly — first a practice of prophecy — became demonized and then trivialized in Western culture.

Seems like my belly has something to say. Excuse me for a moment while I check in. . . .

PANDORA'S BOX

Belly, is there something you want to say?

Tell them there's nothing to fear. Tell them the story of Pandora's box.

Will you tell it with me?

You start, and I'll chime in.

As we hear it these days, *Pandora's box* means something that lets all manner of hell break loose when you look into it. Trouble, hardship, problems, and difficulties all rise up and come at you. You wish you'd never broached the subject, never opened the box to begin with. The story of Pandora's box, as recorded by the Greek poet Hesiod in the eighth century B.C.E., goes like this:

Zeus gave Pandora, a mortal woman, to Prometheus to be his wife. As a wedding gift, Zeus and his buddies gave Pandora a beautiful box and told her not to open it.

What a setup!

Pandora opened the box anyway. Out flew war, pestilence, famine — all the ills and evils besetting humankind. She couldn't shut the lid fast enough to stop them from escaping. But one thing remained at the bottom of the box. What remained was hope.

Pretty wimpy.

As you see, this story blames women for all the troubles of the world.

What a low blow.

You said it.

What's the story on this story?

The story as we know it actually contains an error in translation. When Erasmus was translating the text from Greek into Latin in the sixteenth century, he took the word *pithos*, meaning "vase," for the word *pyxis*, meaning "box." Pandora's vase became Pandora's box.[8]

What's important about that?

For ages, the vase has been a symbol of woman's womb, the belly's capacity for birth and regeneration. Pandora was not a ditz. Nor was she a mortal. *Pandora*, meaning "All-Giver," was another name for Rhea, Great Goddess, Mother of the Universe — the Power of Being imaged in female form.

"Pandora's box" was originally Rhea's vase, meaning her womb. Rhea's vase signified the source of all life.

The story of Pandora's box is one example of Western culture's way of demeaning women and our body's center. The story devalues the womanly belly, taking it from sacred to shameful.

A woman's belly is not Pandora's box!

A woman's belly is Rhea's vase. There's nothing to be afraid of or ashamed of with respect to our bellies. We have every reason to feel proud. Our bellies are awesome.

Yes!

Chapter Three

What's In a Belly?

Your belly is central to your physical health, your emotional well-being, and the flow of vital energy through your body. As you explore the belly in each of these dimensions — physical, emotional, and energetic — you'll discover how these dimensions interweave within the belly as well. You'll see how enlivening your belly with awareness, breath, and movement rejuvenates all of who you are. In this chapter let's focus on the physical.

TAKE THE TOUR: THE PHYSICAL DIMENSION

Come take a tour of the interior. Don't worry — you won't have to tangle with the kind of anatomy that may have bored you in biology class. You won't have to pretend your body is a collection of mechanical pouches, tubes, pumps, and gears. Instead, you'll meet the cast of characters who support your starring role in the adventure of your life. They're some of your best friends, your most dedicated allies.

The purpose of this tour? To reveal ample reason to appreciate your belly and the many ways in which it serves you. (If you want to forgo the details for now, skip to the summary at the end of the chapter, picking up the Perineal Squeeze and your ticket to mindful eating, Eat in Peace, on your way.)

Let's define the territory. Consider the belly to be the region extending from your diaphragm, the broad muscle at the base of your ribs, all the way to your perineum, at the lowest reaches of your torso. For our purposes, we'll include the whole volume of your central body from back to front. Your belly envelops all of your vital organs except for your lungs, your heart, and your brain (and even these organs depend on your belly for their — meaning your — survival).

Skeleton Key: Lovely in Your Bones

Your bones provide stability, structure, and support. The primary bony structure within your belly is your pelvis; the word *pelvis* means "basin" in Latin. Your bowl-shaped pelvis contains and protects your digestive and reproductive organs. During pregnancy, it supports the weight of the developing fetus and provides the passage from womb to world.

Your pelvis mediates the upper and lower regions of your body. The base of your spine — the triangular bone called the sacrum, together with the slender coccyx, or tailbone — inserts into the back of your pelvis, constituting the back of the bowl. Your spine's five lumbar vertebrae rise in a shock-absorbing curve from your sacrum through your lower back, in turn supporting the vertebrae ascending through your chest and neck. Your pelvis's cup-shaped sockets receive the rounded tops of your thighbones, forming your hip joints. These joints anchor your legs, allowing them to rotate, stride, and dance you around town.

Movers and Shakers: Your Muscles

Your abdominal muscles contain your vital organs, position your pelvis, facilitate your breathing, and move your torso. The outermost muscles of your abdominal wall come in pairs: the external and internal obliques, which run diagonally from your ribs to the top ridges of your pelvis. Their fibers orient to each other at right angles. These muscles twist your torso.

Underlying the obliques is the rectus abdominis, running from your lower ribs and the base of your breastbone to your pubic bone. (The parallel bands of connective tissue that cross the rectus abdominis, dividing it into segments, give this muscle its "six-pack" look when it is well toned.) When this muscle contracts, it curls your torso forward.

The deepest layer of muscle in your abdominal wall is the transversus abdominis. Its fibers run perpendicular to those of the rectus abdominis.

All these muscles making up your abdominal wall compress the belly when they contract; when they relax, they allow the belly to expand. If they remain rigid, they restrict your breathing, diminishing your vitality. When they are resilient, they enable you to breathe fully and deeply. At the same time, they hold your vital organs securely in place.

Other muscles deep within your belly both support your spine and equip it to bend forward, backward, and from side to side. The paired psoas muscles, for example, flank your spinal column. They attach to the lumbar vertebrae and run down the length of your pelvis and across your hip joints to insert into the tops of your thighbones.

Performed incorrectly, the sit-ups and ab crunches you might do to flatten your belly can actually overtrain the psoas muscles instead. When these muscles shorten, they tip the top rim of your

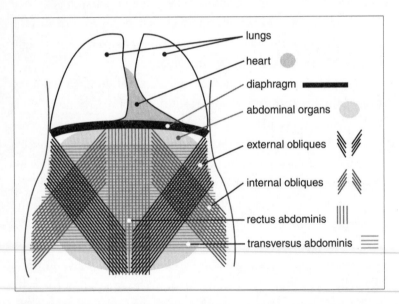

Muscles of the abdominal wall

pelvis forward, spilling your organs forward against your abdominal wall. With your lower back arched and the upper rim of your pelvis thrust forward, your belly sticks out even more than before.

When toned but not habitually tight, the muscles in and around your belly integrate and balance your standing in the world. They animate your journey through life.

A Breath of Fresh Air: Your Organs of Respiration

Your belly's upper border is your respiratory diaphragm, the broad muscle lying at the base of your lungs. Your diaphragm attaches to your ribs and your lumbar spine. It rests directly on your stomach, liver, and spleen, which in turn rest on your small and large intestines.

Respiration is the cycle of taking oxygen in and ushering carbon dioxide out. You need oxygen in abundant, constant supply; deprive the brain of oxygen for even a few minutes, and it begins to die. Inhaling is the way you take in oxygen to fuel your life fire. Exhaling is the way you release carbon dioxide, one of the by-products of combustion, to keep the fire going.

Inhalation occurs as your diaphragm contracts, flattening and descending, increasing the volume of your chest and decreasing the air pressure in and around your lungs relative to the atmosphere outside your body. The partial vacuum occurring in your chest invites air to enter your lungs. Your body receives the oxygen that every cell, tissue, and organ requires. You're literally inspired.

Exhalation takes place as your diaphragm relaxes and rises. Your diaphragm's ascent decreases the volume of your chest, increasing the air pressure in your lungs compared to the air pressure outside your body. Again drawn by the pressure differential, air exits your lungs and takes carbon dioxide out with it as it goes. If allowed to accumulate, such waste products would become toxic and you would expire.

WHAT IS HYPERVENTILATION?

Hyperventilation is rapid, irregular breathing that occurs in the chest and among the ribs. The diaphragm and belly remain relatively immobile. Hyperventilation is a common sign of shock in medical emergencies; it's also frequently a symptom of chronic disorders such as asthma, high blood pressure, ulcers, heart disease, and intestinal inflammation.

Changing the blood's chemistry, hyperventilation reduces the amount of oxygen supplying all the body's tissues, including the brain. Altering the blood's acid-base balance and making it more alkaline, hyperventilation oversensitizes the nervous system and switches on the fight-or-flight response.

In contrast, abdominal breathing delivers generous supplies of oxygen to the body and brain; it signals the nerves and muscles to relax. In a few situations, though, hyperventilation can serve as the body's adaptive balancing act. Disorders such as hypoglycemia, diabetes, and kidney failure, for example, increase the blood's acidity. In such cases, hyperventilation helps restore the blood's original acid-base balance.[1]

The particulars of your breathing affect more than your physical health. The rhythm and range of your diaphragm's movement
determine the depth and quality of your breathing, which
in turn affect your emotional well-being. Short, shallow,
rapid breathing corresponds to feeling rushed, frus-   When I
trated, anxious, fearful, stressed out. Long, deep, slow   breathe, I feel.
breathing corresponds to feeling calm, centered, alert,   — Elaine
relaxed.

Full, deep breathing depends on the muscles in your abdominal wall working in partnership with your diaphragm. If the
muscles of your abdominal wall are resilient — toned but not tight
— they'll expand to make room for your organs moving downward
and outward as your diaphragm descends with your inhalation.
Likewise, if the muscles of your abdominal wall are toned but not
tight, they'll retract and press your organs inward and upward as
your diaphragm ascends with your exhalation. Your inhalation
will be full, and your exhalation will be complete. What could be
more refreshing?

Let's Eat!: Your Organs of Digestion

Your digestive organs break down the food you eat into nutrients
that your body can use for growth and repair. After extracting and
absorbing these nutrients, your digestive organs send them on for
storage and circulation throughout your body. Every tissue in
your body, every way in which your body functions, depends for
sustenance on the digestive organs your belly shelters.

Remember a time when you went without food for a while.
Perhaps you missed a meal or two. How did you feel? Did you get

tired and grumpy? How did you feel after you ate something nourishing? What made the difference?

Your belly, through its capacity for digestion, transforms food into life energy. We can take that for granted, but actually it's quite an achievement. Your digestive organs form one continuous path from inlet to outlet — nearly thirty feet from your mouth to your anus. This long channel provides the ample surface area required for assimilating the nutrients and water that your body needs.

THE VERBAL BODY AND THE EMBODIED WORD

What do the following expressions mean? When, if ever, do you use them? What's their significance for your body? What other examples of "body language" have you heard?

I can't stomach this,
I've got butterflies in my
    stomach.
That makes me sick to my
    stomach.
My stomach is tied up in
    knots.
I'm scared shitless.
I've got the runs.
I feel shitty.
I'm pissed.
I'm fed up.

That's hard to swallow.
I've had a bellyful.
That galls me.
I need to vent my spleen.
I need to air my feelings.
I'm being lily-livered.
I'm starving for attention.
They hate my guts.
It's gut-wrenching.
My gut reaction is...
I've got a gut feeling.
I'll go with my gut.

Your Stomach

Your stomach is the crescent-shaped organ on the left side of your body positioned just under your diaphragm. Empty, its volume is about two cups; it can expand by a factor of four to hold as much as two quarts of food.

With a wavelike, churning motion of its muscular wall, your stomach breaks down the food you eat physically as well as chemically; it processes more than one thousand pounds of food annually. In a seventy-year life span, a stomach digests more than thirty-three tons of food.

Your stomach secretes about two quarts of gastric enzymes and hydrochloric acid daily. This hydrochloric acid is strong enough to burn a hole in a wool carpet. Constituting 0.5 percent of your stomach's digestive juices, it enhances your immunity by neutralizing agents of disease. It also corrodes the esophagus, gums, and teeth of women who, caught in the binge-and-purge cycle of the eating disorder known as bulimia, repeatedly vomit their food to avoid digesting it.

Your Small Intestine

Your small intestine, about seventeen feet long, proceeds from your stomach and packs itself in twists and S-curves into the center of your belly. The small intestine receives partially digested food from your stomach and shreds it further with muscular agitation and enzyme action, completing the extraction and absorption of nutrients within its length.

The inner lining of your small intestine is folded into thousands of finger-shaped protrusions, called villi, which remove nutrients from food and distribute them to the body's tissues. The villi effectively increase the surface area of your small intestine's lining by a factor of ten thousand. If this lining were stretched out flat, it would be the size of a tennis court.

Your Large Intestine

Undigested remnants of food pass from your small intestine into your large intestine, also known as the colon or bowel. The large intestine makes one 5-foot loop around the coil of your small intestine, ascending along the right side of your belly, continuing across to your left side at the lower border of your ribs, and descending along your left side. Your colon then curves back toward your body's midline, becoming your rectum. Your digestive tract ends with your anal opening.

Your rectum collects and stores fecal matter. Elimination occurs when the wavelike motion of your colon's muscular lining combines with the relaxation of the muscles ringing your anal opening and the voluntary contraction of your abdominal muscles. This joint action moves feces from your rectum out through your anal canal.

Constipation signals a disturbance in the process of elimination. Overuse and abuse of laxatives can contribute to constipation by overriding the body's own impulses for defecation.

Your Liver, Gallbladder, and Pancreas

Your liver, gallbladder, and pancreas collaborate with the organs of your digestive tract. The liver is your body's largest organ, weighing about three pounds. Situated on the right side of your body directly under your diaphragm, it extends from midchest down to the border of your ribs.

WHAT MAKES A BELLY GROWL?

The rumbles, gurgles, and growls your belly makes mark the progress of peristalsis, the wavelike action of your digestive tract's muscular walls. Peristalsis propels the food that's being digested through your stomach and small intestine, moves the remaining indigestible matter through your large intestine, and expels these remnants when you defecate.

Peristalsis is subject to the nervous system's interaction with the digestive organs. Signals from the nerves are likely to turn peristalsis off in situations of stress and turn it on again when the stress diminishes. Accordingly, the bowel sounds you hear may correspond to your body's shift from a state of stress into a state of greater relaxation.

My belly often gurgles when I'm dialoguing with it in writing. In fact, it gets particularly vocal right when I've found my way to articulating the truth of the matter. (It just growled!) Bowel sounds and truth-telling occur together so frequently that I suspect there's a significant connection. I suspect that saying what I mean at the deepest level — being authentic — (my belly's making *lots* of sounds now!) produces a kind of bodily sigh, a relaxation that promotes peristalsis and an affirmative rumbling in my gut.

Your liver performs many functions, including processing and storing the nutrients absorbed by your small and large intestines, processing carbohydrates into simple sugars for immediate energy use, and removing toxins and neutralizing poisons, such as alcohol and drugs. Your liver also makes as much as one quart of bile daily to assist the digestion of fats taking place in your small intestine.

Your gallbladder is a pear-shaped sac, about four inches long, sitting in an indentation on the underside of your liver's right lobe. It stores the bile that your liver produces, releasing this thick, yellow-green liquid into your small intestine to digest fats.

Resting to the left of your liver and tucked behind your stomach is your pancreas. This slender, triangular gland, six inches long, produces more than a quart of digestive enzymes daily, supplying them directly to your small intestine. It also makes insulin and glucagon, two hormones that circulate throughout your body and regulate cellular energy use.

Eat in Peace

Your belly's digestive organs turn food into the fuel that keeps you alive. They transform what you eat into the substance of who you are — bone, muscle, blood, skin, and all the other tissues that comprise your physical self. When you eat in peace, you give your belly the time and place it needs to do this vital work for you. Some women have found that their bodies shed excess weight when they attend to eating with gratitude and self-respect.

Rushing through what you're eating can make your belly grumble with indignation — indigestion, that is. Taking the time to notice what you're eating helps develop your intuitive sense of what nourishes your body best. As your inner guidance becomes clear, it's easier to choose the foods that suit your individual needs, no matter what diet program may be in fashion.

Slowing down the process of eating means chewing thoroughly. Chewing your food well gets your digestion off to a good start, giving your body the nutrients it needs and promoting swift elimination.

Giving yourself a peaceful setting in which to eat enables you to distinguish hunger for food from other needs. When you're distracted, you can easily mistake many feelings — anger, fear, excitement, boredom, fatigue, sadness — for hunger. Focusing your attention allows you to know what and how much you need to truly satisfy yourself.

EAT IN PEACE

Begin by eating one meal or snack in peace each week. Make it a special treat!

1. Set aside ample time for preparing food, cleaning up, and then relaxing after you eat.

2. Slow down. Notice the colors and textures of the food you're preparing. Consider how this food has come into your hands. How many people and resources have played a part in bringing it to you?

3. Create a peaceful setting. Add a touch of beauty to your table with a picture, flower, candle, special bowl, soothing

music — whatever pleases you. Turn off the radio or television. Sit down to eat. If you're eating with others, make an
agreement to keep conversation simple and pleasant. Arrange
to address problems and conflicts after the meal.

4. Enter into the Centering Breath. Notice the sensations oc-
    curring in your belly. How do you experience being hungry?

5. Regard the food on your plate as a gift. Savor its color,
    shape, texture. Bring the food toward your mouth and, even
    before you taste it, enjoy its aroma.

6. Place the food in your mouth, then put down your fork or
    spoon. Enjoy the temperature, texture, and density of the
    food in your mouth. Begin chewing.

7. As you chew, notice the strength of your jaw muscles, the
    motion of your tongue and lips. Notice how chewing re-
    leases the food's flavors. Enjoy the taste. How many flavors
    do you taste?

8. Chew until you've liquefied the food. As you swallow, feel
    your body receiving nourishment.

9. Notice sensations in your belly and your degree of hunger
    now. Are you ready for another bite?

10. Take a few moments at the end of your meal to appreciate
    the nourishment that you've created and received.

BLUEBERRY MUFFIN REUNION

Blueberries are angels' beads unstrung;
you're the messenger that brings these gems
to me. Others may fear you, counting

your calories, grams of fat, label you
bad. I don't. You beckoned to me from
the bakery's bin, promised to please me,
feed my hunger. The hands that planted
and milled the wheat, harvested salt,
pressed the oil, stirred the batter and
filled the tins raise their palms to me
in benediction. You have gone through flood
of milk and oven's fire for me. And now
we meet: what's offered, what's received.

In the alchemy of ovens you have risen.
Whatever I have muffed is well-forgiven.

Making Babies (or Not): Your Organs of Reproduction

Your reproductive organs bear the capacity to generate new life, to egg on creation. From menarche, your first menstrual cycle, to menopause, your menstrual cycle regulates the maturation of egg cells and prepares your uterus to support fetal development.

The outermost structure of your reproductive system is your vulva. Within your vulva's outer and inner lips are the openings to your vagina and to your urethra, which leads to your bladder. The vulva also shelters your clitoris, the only structure within your body whose sole function is to provide pleasure. The oval shape of the vaginal opening figures in the sacred symbols of many cultures. The Egyptian *ankh*, for example, features an oval atop a cross. It signifies the capacity for rebirth and eternal life.

Your vagina leads from your vulva to the cervix at the base of your pear-shaped, muscular uterus. The small central opening of the cervix leads into the uterine interior. Except during pregnancy, your uterus is about the size of a fist — three inches long, two inches wide.

Extending right and left from your uterus are uterine tubes. (They're also called Fallopian tubes but, with all due respect, these body parts don't belong to Dr. Gabriele Fallopio, the Italian surgeon who named them in the sixteenth century.) Each of these curving channels is about five inches long and ends in fingerlike projections adjacent to each ovary. Your almond-shaped ovaries are each about two inches long and one inch wide.

I no longer feel that I have a knife in my belly. If I ask my belly what it wants to eat for lunch and I eat that, it doesn't hurt. My belly's the first place where tension shows up. If my stomach is hurting, it's letting me know that something has happened that's upset me.

— *Martha*

At puberty, each of your ovaries contains about two hundred thousand prototypical egg cells. Following menarche, your ovaries stimulate egg cells to mature into ova. In the process, they secrete the hormones — estrogen and progesterone — that time the phases of menstruation, the monthly bleeding that is menses.

Menses is a Latin word meaning "months," signifying that the length of the menstrual cycle is often twenty-eight days, the interval of the lunar month. The Sanskrit word for women's monthly cycle of bleeding is *rtü*, the root of the word *ritual*.[2] This association suggests that our menstrual cycle is the origin of humankind's intimate, recurring relationship with the sacred.

Contemporary Western culture generally considers a woman's menstrual period as something unclean, something that's best ignored. In other times and cultures, though, women have known their monthly, moon-wise periods of bleeding to be a special time for renewal, secluding themselves in a hut or tent apart from the rest of the clan.

Your Perineum

Your belly's lower border is your perineum, two triangles joined together to form a diamond-shaped field. The forward section, the urogenital triangle, supports your clitoris, urethral opening, and vaginal opening. Positioned above and to the rear of the urogenital triangle is the anal triangle; its levator ani muscle forms your pelvic floor, also called the pelvic diaphragm.

Your perineum holds your vagina, uterus, and bladder in position. Strengthening this muscular foundation — which can lose tone with childbirth and menopause — prevents and alleviates uterine prolapse and urinary incontinence.

A portion of the pelvic diaphragm, the pubococcygeal (PC) muscle, runs from your pubic bone to your coccyx, enclosing your vagina. Since orgasm occurs with repeated contractions of the PC muscle, strengthening the PC muscle increases the intensity of orgasm.

When the PC muscle and the muscles of your lower abdomen contract at the same time, your uterus lifts and flattens, opening the area at the top of the vagina that lies underneath, and is usually closed off by, the uterus. This area is richly supplied with nerve endings. Making it available to stimulation magnifies the pleasure of orgasm.

THE PERINEAL SQUEEZE

The Perineal Squeeze is an effective exercise for strengthening your PC muscle and your entire pelvic floor. A strong pelvic floor keeps your uterus and bladder in place and helps to prevent prolapse. Toning the muscles of your pelvic floor also eliminates incontinence, enabling you to laugh, cough, jump, and run without fear of wetting yourself. Before, during, and after pregnancy, such toning prepares and restores the pelvic muscles engaged during childbirth.

I.   Lie on your back, your arms at your sides and your legs extending straight out from your hips. Cross your right ankle over the left. Inhale fully.

2.   Exhale and tilt your pelvis to lengthen your lower back, gently pressing the back of your waist into the ground. With your head remaining on the ground, gently press your chin down toward your chest, lengthening the back of your neck.

     At the same time, press your thighs and buttocks together and contract the muscles around your anal opening. Contract the muscles of your vaginal wall, tightening high up inside your vagina. Squeeze and lift all these muscles in and up toward your belly center.

3.   With your breath still held out, continue squeezing and lifting for five to ten seconds. Then, as you inhale, release your vagina and perineum fully; relax your entire body. Repeat as many as ten times. Feel what's happening in your body.

4.   Reverse the position of your legs, crossing your left ankle over the right, and repeat, as many as ten times. Again, feel what's happening in your body.

Notes:

◉   To avoid interrupting the discharge of blood, do not prac-
    tice the Perineal Squeeze during heavy menstrual flow.

◉   To avoid raising your blood pressure, be sure to hold your
    breath *out* as you hold the contraction; release the squeeze
    as you inhale.

◉   To relieve urinary incontinence, practice the Perineal Squeeze
    frequently — for example, ten repetitions three times a day,
    holding each squeeze for ten seconds.

◉   As a preparation for childbirth (in consultation with your
    health care provider), practice the Perineal Squeeze frequently
    — for example, for as long as two minutes every two hours
    throughout the day.

◉   Once you're familiar with the process, you can practice the
    Perineal Squeeze (without crossing your ankles) when you're
    standing and sitting as well. In this variation, simply focus
    on the way your pubic bone and tailbone move toward each
    other as you lift your perineum up toward your belly center
    with each exhalation.

Pregnancy

Pregnancy occurs when an ovum receives a sperm, is fertilized, and then attaches to the uterine wall. As the fertilized egg develops into an embryo and then a fetus, its point of attachment
becomes the umbilical cord, the conduit transporting oxygen and
nutrients from woman to fetus as well as removing fetal wastes.

The surrounding uterus protects the developing fetus and accommodates its growth. Originally the size of a fist, it expands to fill the entire abdomen.

At birth, uterine contractions push the fetus out through the vagina. After the baby is born and the umbilical cord is clamped and cut, the opening to the baby's belly closes. The stump of the umbilical cord eventually dries and falls off, and the umbilicus — otherwise known as the navel or belly button — remains. Following childbirth, a woman's vagina and uterus retract to nearly their previous dimensions.

WHAT MAKES A BELLY BUTTON?

One woman calls her navel her first scar, her "mother-scar." If our navels could talk, they might tell us how we're still connected to our mothers.

How are you still connected to your mother? Media artist Judith Selby filmed women and men answering that question while baring their midriffs to the camera. Only their midsections are visible onscreen. As you hear these people's words, all you see is their belly buttons moving. Their navels are speaking indeed![3]

The belly button marks something we all have in common. Whatever our gender, race, creed, ethnicity, or national origin, our human origin is the same: we are all born by women. Before other attributes and allegiances, we were first citizens of the womb-world. We each bear the mother-scar to remind us of our beginnings in a woman's belly.

In the Flow: Your Organs of Circulation and Excretion

As it flows through your body, blood distributes oxygen, nutrients, immune agents, and hormones to the body's cells and tissues; it carries away the wastes and toxins that, if they accumulate, contribute to disease.

Your heart pumps oxygenated, nutrient-rich blood into your body through a branching network of arteries. Blood returns from your body's cells and tissues to your heart through a complementary network of veins.

But your heart is not on its own in moving blood through your body. The blood returning to your heart from your legs and abdomen must rise against gravity. Expanding and contracting your abdominal muscles helps out your heart by pumping the venous blood upward. When your belly moves with your breath, it actively participates in circulating your blood.

Blood is not the only fluid of note. Your organs of excretion — kidneys, ureters, bladder, and urethra — filter your blood and discharge waste products as urine.

Your kidneys are each about four inches long and flank the upper reaches of your lumbar spine, resting behind your liver, stomach, and large intestine. Each of your kidneys contains more than one million filtering components, called nephrons. They remove waste from your blood and also adjust the volume and content of your bodily fluids.

A pair of ureters conducts urine from your kidneys down to storage in your bladder, situated in front of and under your uterus. Urine passes out from your bladder through your urethra.

Your perineum supports your urethra and helps to hold your

bladder in place. Strengthening the perineal muscles with the Perineal Squeeze helps to prevent your bladder from leaking.

Homeland Security: Your Organs of Immunity

Your abdominal organs contribute to your immunity in a number of ways. Your stomach, for example, secretes acids and enzymes, helping to eliminate the agents of disease that might enter your body with what you eat and drink. Your liver actively neutralizes and removes toxins. The nerves embedded in the lining of your digestive tract secrete small protein molecules named peptides, which can stimulate your immune response.

Your belly plays a major role in your lymph system. This complex network of elements includes lymph fluid, specialized cells called lymphocytes, lymph organs, nodes, and vessels. Your lymph system extends immunity throughout your body by flushing agents of disease out of your cells and neutralizing them.

> My husband is a paramedic. He works on an ambulance and brings home every virus imaginable. He gets sick. I don't. I do my belly exercises.
>
> — *Teresa*

Your spleen, resting directly under your diaphragm on the left side of your belly behind your stomach, is your body's largest lymphatic organ. Your spleen stores lymphocytes and filters your blood, removing defective blood cells and agents of disease that have been circulating in your blood.

The lining of your digestive tract includes lymphatic nodules, dense clusters of lymphocytes; the membranes that enclose your digestive organs include lymph vessels and nodes as well. These nodes and nodules are poised to inactivate the pathogens you may have ingested along with your food and water.

WHAT IS A BELLY LAUGH?

In his encounter with a painful disease — degeneration of the connective tissue in his spine and joints — author Norman Cousins discovered the healing power of laughter. He found healing in belly laughter — great, gutsy guffaws, that is, not timid tee-hees.

Cousins designed his treatment to include watching outrageous Marx Brothers movies and *Candid Camera* reruns. He found that ten minutes of side-splitting laughter provided enough pain relief to allow him at least two hours of revitalizing sleep. Blood tests confirmed that the cumulative improvements in his health lasted long after his bouts of belly laughing.

Other research documents that laughter boosts immunity, decreases blood pressure, and reduces the incidence of hormones associated with stress. It may guard against heart disease. Laughing a hundred times gives you the equivalent of ten to fifteen minutes' worth of cardiovascular exercise.

What provokes your belly laughter? Perhaps you get a glimpse of what's both absurd and profound, chaotic and orderly, mundane and mystical, tawdry and glorious.

What is a belly laugh? It's aerobics for your innards. It's the quiver your body makes as outmoded concepts crackle and rigid certainties crumble. It's the shiver your body makes as tension dissolves, as you open to the present moment and reap the great relief: returning, once again, to your center.

The lymph fluid that has flushed your digestive organs, your urinary and reproductive organs, and the tissues of your legs flows through your belly's network of lymph vessels and collects in major conduits. From your belly, the lymph rises through your chest to merge with venous blood and return to your heart.

Lymph fluid has no pump of its own to push it up from your legs and lower body against the pull of gravity. The lymph moving through your belly and returning to your heart depends on rhythmical muscular action for its circulation. Expanding and contracting your abdominal muscles — as you do when you practice the belly-energizing exercises presented in part 2 — pumps your lymph fluid through your belly's network of vessels, actively enhancing your immunity to disease.

Some Nerve: Your Organs of Perception and Stimulation

Your central nervous system includes your brain and your spinal cord, extending through the core of your body into your belly. Spinal nerves branch out from your spinal cord and subdivide, generating a network of nerves that reaches through the volume of your body and out to your body's periphery, regulating the action of muscles, organs, and glands. A portion of this peripheral organization of nerves is largely involuntary, or autonomic — subject to unconscious rather than conscious direction.

This autonomic nerve network includes complementary systems called the sympathetic and parasympathetic divisions. By participating in the process of breathing, your belly interacts with both of these divisions and helps to determine the degree to which you feel stressed or relaxed.

The nerves of your sympathetic system engage your body's fight-or-flight response to stress. The sympathetic nerves move blood from your visceral organs to your skeletal muscles, equipping them for action. These nerves also reduce peristalsis and slow digestion, increasing your heart and breathing rates as well.

When your sympathetic system is engaged, your breathing is short, rapid, and shallow. Such breathing takes place high in your chest, leaving your belly isolated and immobile. The same is true in reverse: short, rapid, shallow breathing activates your sympathetic system and invokes the stress response.

The parasympathetic division of your autonomic nervous system balances the action of the sympathetic nerves. The nerves of the parasympathetic division promote your body's relaxation response, relieving stress.

The parasympathetic nerves move blood from your skeletal muscles back to your abdominal organs, increasing peristalsis and enhancing digestion, and also reducing your heart and breathing rates. When your parasympathetic system is engaged, you feel calm, content, and sexually expressive.

When your parasympathetic nervous system is active, your breathing is long, slow, and deep; your belly participates in your breathing, moving rhythmically toward and away from your spine in the steady cycle of your exhalation and inhalation. The same is true in reverse: when your breathing is long, slow, and deep, with your belly serving as a bellows for the breath — as in the Centering Breath — you engage your parasympathetic system and invoke the relaxation response.

Another component of your nervous system is the enteric nervous system — ENS for short. Located within the muscles lining your gut, the ENS is rapidly gaining repute as a "second brain." This network of nerves maintains two-way communication with the brain that's housed in the skull. It can also learn and operate quite independently. The ENS mediates our physical and emotional experience, giving substance to the term "gut feeling." The next chapter addresses this subject in more detail.

THE BOTTOM LINE

When you allow your belly to move out and in as you inhale and exhale, you're realizing your capacity to breathe deeply. You're giving your body and brain the generous supply of oxygen they need. You're equipping yourself to be healthy and happy.

If you suck in your abs or your clothes are so tight that they make your middle rigid, you cut your belly out of the loop. Then all you can do is sniff at the air with your nose, shoulders, and chest. That's a sure recipe for building up tension and anxiety. Such shallow breathing reduces the supply of oxygen to your body and brain. The way your nerves are wired, shallow breathing automatically makes you feel stressed. Is that what you want?

LAUREL'S STORY

Your abdominal muscles and the clothes you wear determine how freely your diaphragm can move and how fully you can breathe. If your abdomen is rigid, it restricts your diaphragm and makes your breathing shallow, increasing your sense of stress. When your abdominal muscles are toned but not tight, your diaphragm is free to move and deepen your breathing, increasing your sense of self-assurance.

"I want to breathe more deeply," one woman told me; I'll call her Laurel to respect her privacy. "My breath is shallow; it stays up in my chest. Since I was little, I've been taught to hold my stomach in. My mother was very concerned about her figure, and as a child I picked up on that. Can you help me learn how to breathe more deeply?" Here's how Laurel discovered the connection between her breath and her self-esteem:

I suggested we begin with a meditation and invited Laurel to explore whatever images might emerge in the region of her belly. On completing the meditation, she told me, "I saw a thick blue-gray band wrapping around my belly. That band keeps me from breathing fully. It keeps me from connecting to people."

"Can you remember a time when you *were* breathing deeply?" I asked.

Instantly, she recalled, "Until I was five or six, my family lived on a farm. I didn't have the band around my stomach then. We lived next door to my grandparents. We lived out in the country, so I didn't have anyone else to play with. I was close to my grandparents, saw them every day. I was especially close to my grandfather. It was paradise.

"So it tore me up when we moved to town. I didn't have any friends, didn't know how to make friends. One day, after we'd moved, I was walking through the neighborhood behind my sister, Jill. She was four years older than me and seemed like an adult to me; I worshipped her. She turned around and made a gesture like she was going to kill me. 'Leave me alone!' she shouted. 'I'm going to make friends, and I don't want you to come with me.' I ran home and cried. I didn't know how to make friends, and my big sister wouldn't show me how. That's when my breath became shallow. I became a worrier, anxious."

I guided Laurel into the Centering Breath, inviting her to place her hands on her lower abdomen and imagine a beautiful balloon inside her belly that filled with the incoming breath and emptied with the outgoing breath. As she did so, I asked her to simply watch what happened to the band, without trying to change it in any way. As she continued breathing and watching, she told me that the band was becoming thinner and broader, more resilient; it changed in color from a dull blue-gray to a translucent blue and then to a blue-white luminescence.

We followed the Centering Breath with some belly-energizing exercises, using these power-centering moves not only to deepen the breath and dissolve tension in the abdomen but also to enact gestures of affirmation. For example, as Laurel moved through the Lily (see pages 194–96), with her arms spread wide, she was making this statement to her sister and to the world: "I am *here*. I am claiming my right to be noticed, included, and valued."

As we concluded our time together, Laurel commented, "I can breathe deeply now. And I'm feeling I can make connections with other people." Her renewed self-confidence and her readiness to connect with others demonstrated the immediate benefits she received in activating her *hara*.

This woman, who'd been schooled since childhood to flatten her stomach, also made the link between breathing deeply and allowing her belly to take its natural shape. As we were parting, she said, "I've seen pictures of African women with nice round bellies. They look so healthy. Is there anything like that for Western women?"

Expanding and contracting your belly with the breath strengthens your abdominal muscles in a balanced way. Belly breathing also allows all the organs housed within your belly to work for you at peak performance. Containing the organs that are vital to your life, your belly is your best friend for calming your nerves, improving your digestion and elimination, enhancing your circulation, boosting your immunity, revitalizing your reproductive organs, and magnifying your sexual pleasure. What's not to love?

Chapter Four

Secrets of
Your Body's Center

Now let's explore the emotional and energetic life of the body's center. The reward? Access to a wealth of creative power and healing wisdom that you might otherwise miss.

BUTTERFLIES IN YOUR STOMACH:
THE EMOTIONAL DIMENSION

Although we can speak of *mind* and *body* as if we were describing separate items, are they really so distinct? Thoughts, emotions, and physical experience overlap and intertwine. The mind-belly connection is especially intimate.

Physiological events can alter emotions; emotions translate into physiological events. A "gut-wrenching" experience, for example, can involve both anguish in your mind and aching in your belly.

What's your experience? How perky do you feel when you're constipated? How playful do you feel when you've got PMS? How confident do you feel when your stomach is tied up in knots?

If you've been down in the dumps, how do you feel after you've taken a brisk walk? You may have already discovered that belly-energizing movement and breathing can improve your mood.

The previous chapter revealed how the belly is connected to the nervous system's setup for stress and relaxation. It also detailed the belly's role in helping you breathe deeply, infusing your body and brain with adequate supplies of oxygen. Clinical research shows that regular oxygen-enhancing exercise can be as effective a treatment for depression as an antidepressant drug.[1] Imagine a psychiatrist's prescription pad with the notation, *Give yourself room to breathe. Breathe deeply.*

That would be a powerful prescription. For you to breathe deeply, the muscular dome of your diaphragm must be resilient, free to move. If the diaphragm is constantly tense, it becomes immobile. Then the body has to struggle to breathe, using muscles in the chest and between the ribs. The shallow, rapid pattern of breath that results deprives the brain of oxygen, only increasing the sense of anxiety or despair.

The diaphragm tenses when we try to put a lid on our feelings. This broad muscle at the base of the lungs clenches when we attempt to ignore the emotions — such as grief, anger, and rage — that typically come to a boil in the belly below. But denying emotions doesn't make them go away. As aggravating as this insight may be, resisting the sensations we'd rather not feel turns pain into something more — suffering.

Although denial may have some short-term appeal, it's not necessarily a permanent solution. We invite a more rewarding resolution when we choose to breathe more deeply, allowing the diaphragm to descend and release, allowing the belly to expand and release. Breathing deeply adds one of the necessary ingredients for healing — oxygen — to the mix.

When you breathe more deeply, numbness gives way to sensation. Denial gives way to awareness. When you breathe, you feel. So be gentle with yourself. Go slowly, with respect and with compassion — for yourself and for others. The initial return of awareness may be a bit uncomfortable. Yet as you witness rather than resist sensation, vitality flows again to where it's needed most. Breath and compassionate awareness combine to help relieve emotional distress and resolve the situation from which it has emerged.

> The breathing and belly work dissipated my menstrual cramps this morning. Ahhhhhh.
>
> — Tricia

Still, there's more to your belly's role in managing how you feel. Your belly is home to your reproductive organs, which secrete and circulate hormones such as estrogen and progesterone. When these hormones are out of balance, they can put your emotions on a roller coaster. By stimulating blood flow and dispelling congestion, belly-energizing movement and breathing patterns can help even out the ride.

Smart Belly

As mentioned in chapter 3, your belly is home to a major portion of the nervous system — the enteric nervous system, or ENS — that lines your entire gastrointestinal tract, beginning with your esophagus.

Your "gut brain" and the brain that's up top in your skull, the "cranial brain," are derived from the same embryological tissues and produce the same biochemicals, called neurotransmitters, which turn nerve impulses into physiological action. One such biochemical, which plays a major role in relieving depression, is serotonin. Popular antidepressant drugs, such as Prozac, likely work by maintaining a generous supply of serotonin in the cranial brain.

Your enteric nervous system not only produces serotonin — it produces a lot of it. In fact, your gut produces and stores 95 percent of your body's total supply of serotonin. The serotonin in your gut plays many roles in managing your digestion. It starts the process by stimulating the secretion of enzymes from the pancreas. And it orchestrates the pace and rhythm of peristalsis, the wavelike muscular contractions that move food through your digestive tract.

You may already be aware of the action of serotonin in your belly. Too much or too little of this biochemical speeds up or slows down peristalsis. The result? Diarrhea or constipation.

Your gut brain doesn't share its abundant supply of serotonin with your cranial brain, but its serotonin does influence the cranial brain by stimulating the tenth cranial nerve (also known as the vagus nerve). This nerve descends from the cranial brain stem through the neck to the abdomen, allowing for two-way talk between the gut and cranial brains. The gut is the chatty one, sending up nine nerve impulses for every one it receives in return. Even with all this checking in, the enteric nervous system in the gut can operate largely independently of the cranial brain —

making its own measurements and assessments, initiating its own decisions, and learning its own lessons.

The enteric nervous system also comes into play in conjunction with an immune response that the cranial brain initiates. Here's one possible scenario: When substances threaten to breach the gut's lining — substances including stress hormones, as well as natural and industrial pathogens — the cranial brain activates the immune system's special agents, its mast cells, and appoints them to guard the gut wall. Doing their job, the mast cells secrete biochemicals, such as histamines, that induce inflammation. The inflamed tissues make the enteric nerves overly sensitive and overactive, deregulating the production of serotonin. Chronic inflammation gets on the gut's nerves. It would make anyone irritable.

Although the causes of irritable bowel syndrome (IBS) may not be well understood, many women are familiar with the signs of this functional bowel disorder. Common symptoms include abdominal bloating, cramping, and pain, and sometimes constipation alternating with diarrhea. According to the International Foundation for Functional Gastrointestinal Disorders, this particular kind of misery affects as many as one out of five adults, mostly women. Colitis, Crohn's disease, and other forms of inflammatory bowel disease (IBD) affect many more.

The connection between your mood and how your bowels are moving extends to anxiety and depression. As Dr. Emeran Mayer, director of the Center for Neurovisceral Sciences & Women's Health at the University of California, Los Angeles, asserts, "The majority of patients with anxiety and depression will also have alterations of their GI function."[2] He goes on to reveal that nearly three-quarters of those he has treated for chronic gastrointestinal disorders have suffered severe stresses as children. They've witnessed their parents divorcing, for example. Or they've endured a parent's death. Such events can disrupt the sense of security and connection — the sense of being mothered, being nurtured — that a child needs to digest experience and absorb nourishment throughout her life.

MEDIATING YOUR MIND-BELLY RELATIONSHIP

If you're experiencing distress in your body's center — if you've got a bellyache of one sort or another — the following questions may help you clarify the reciprocal influence of mind and body. (For more ways to reconcile mind and belly, see practices such as Start a Correspondence and Draw Out Your Deepest Knowing in chapters 10 and 11.)

When did this distress start?

What was going on in your life at the time?

What are your symptoms — not in medical terminology but in the actuality of what you feel, see, hear, taste, smell, and intuit?

When do these sensations intensify?

When do these sensations diminish or disappear?

If your symptoms could talk, what would they say?

If this distress were a message that you need to forgive or love yourself more in some way, how might you do that?

Compassionate body awareness, movement, and breath might contribute to healing gastrointestinal distress. How? Since your belly is home to your entire digestive tract except for your esophagus, your belly also encompasses the major portion of your enteric nervous system. When you're energizing your belly, you're interacting with this system of nerves.

As Dr. Michael Gershon, a leading investigator in the expanding field of neurogastroenterology and author of *The Second Brain*, says, "The gut monitors pressure."[3] Here's what I suspect: When you breathe deeply, rhythmically contracting and expanding your belly, you're sending soothing signals to your enteric nerves. You're reducing their arousal. You're singing a lullaby. You're rocking the cradle, ever so gently.

> I've made peace with the fact that I love my mother and I don't like — sometimes hate — her personality. My digestion is better now. I'm cooking more carefully for myself.
>
> — Elizabeth

Core Energy, Core Issues

Our bellies are not mechanical body parts. Like us, they're alive. Like us, they are sentient — caring, feeling, knowing, discerning — beings. They shelter the pro-creative power concentrated in our body's core.

When the pro-creative power that our bellies embody is denied, repressed, or displaced, we're just not happy. We're irritable. We're angry and inflamed. No matter how hard or fast we try to run from it, there's a bottomless hole at the center of our lives that no external fix — not even shopping — can fill.

SEROTONIN, PERISTALSIS, AND THE ORIGINS OF LIFE

The connections among the enteric nervous system, serotonin production, and peristalsis are currently the subject of much study. At the risk of sending the registrar at the university that awarded me a degree in biology shrieking to the files to revoke my diploma, I offer you the following meditation.

Where did life on this planet begin? In the ocean.

Picture our ancestral life in the sea. It was simple, wasn't it? All we had to do was allow waves of seawater to wash through us and hold on to the nutrients the water carried with it, on the tide.

Okay, maybe we weren't always quite so passive. Maybe we got inventive. Maybe we modified the water's wave action with filaments and threadlike projections. We set up a favorable current for ourselves, directing the incoming nutrients to where we could most easily absorb them.

Fast-forward to the twenty-first century. You still bring nutrients in from the outside. However convoluted your thirty-foot-long digestive tract may be, it's still a channel open to the environment in which you are immersed.

You and the muscles lining your digestive tract are still making wavelike movements to usher nutrients in the appropriate direction. Managing this wavelike process, this peristalsis, is the serotonin that's produced and stored in your gut.

The muscular wave motion that ensures our physical nourishment now replicates the tidal action that fed us back when we dwelled in our original home, Ocean Mother. The rhythmic contraction and release taking place in our digestive tracts also links us to our childhood experiences of being mothered, being nurtured. The divorce, death, or other trauma that ruptures our primal nourishing relationships may also disrupt the production of serotonin and the process of peristalsis, leading to gastrointestinal distress.

What goes on in your gut may well reflect how you have experienced being nourished in several dimensions: in relationship to the food you eat and the water you drink, in relationship to the people who mothered you, and in relationship to Ocean Mother, the totality of life itself.

When our pro-creative power gets stymied, our bellies display corresponding symptoms of physical distress. The signs can range from stomachaches to constipation to fibroids to eating disorders. These are signals that something is blocking the flow of our vital life force. They're indicators that some core issue or issues must be addressed.

When my belly gets bloated, it's asking me to attend more carefully, more conscientiously, to myself. The protrusion demonstrates that I'm projecting myself — my Self — in some way. Now it's time to ask, How am I giving myself and my authority away to someone or something else?

To restart the process of attending to my inner guidance, I need to engage in practices such as Naming Your Feelings and others detailed in part 2, such as Dialogue with Your Inner Wisdom. If I've been giving away my own authority, no amount of following someone else's rules for diet and exercise is going to address the core issue my belly is calling to my attention.

The core issues our bellies demonstrate often relate to:

- Giving, receiving, and absorbing nourishment
- Sorting out and rejecting what is toxic
- Setting boundaries
- Establishing identity
- Releasing the need to be perfect
- Feeling that we're being enough, doing enough, having enough

- Expressing anger
- Living with a sense of purpose
- Voicing the truth
- Affirming sexuality
- Being safe when being sexual
- Expressing creativity
- Living with a sense of abundance
- Grieving and letting go

Mothering and Being Mothered

Many factors contribute to the core issues I've just listed. At the same time, all of them relate to the fundamental challenges of mothering and being mothered.

As mothers, how can we help our daughters grow into self-validating, self-actualizing adults if we've not been nurtured that way ourselves? Unless we invent beliefs and behaviors that reach way beyond what our own experience has taught us, we're likely to train our daughters to carry on traditions of disempowerment.

As daughters, how can we reject the disempowering elements of our mothers' training without rejecting our mothers as well? Unless we respect the limitations and restrictions that our mothers have encountered, we're likely to fray or break our connection with them.

Our core issues correspond to the challenges implicit in our relationship with Mother in every dimension — our biological mothers, Mother Earth, and Mother of the Universe.

BEING MOTHERED

One day a vivid image of being mothered came to my mind. I saw that during the time I was developing in my mother's womb, a blue-rimmed field of golden energy stood behind her. I understood this energy to be Shakti, an Indian name for the Mother of the Universe. I saw this Shakti energy streaming into my mother's body through a point in the center of her lower back and filling her belly. The Shakti energy likewise infused me as my mother's belly sheltered me and then birthed me out into the world. I understood that in giving birth to me, my mother had allowed her body to be a vessel for the Great Mother.

In the years following this vision, I learned that the point in my mother's back that I saw opening to receive Shakti energy is called *mingmen*, or "Life Gate," in the Asian healing arts. Complementing the belly center, it is the point of entry for Source Energy. I also learned that, in Egyptian tradition, the universal soul attending the individual soul at birth and death is called *Ka*, and her benediction is "Behold, I am behind thee, I am thy temple, thy mother, forever and forever."

Our bellies are our connection to our mothers, to the women who held us in their bellies, birthed us into the world, and nurtured us to the best of their ability. Our bellies, sheltering our pro-creative power, are also our connection to the Power of Being that nurtures and sustains our lives and the world at large.

Whatever our mothers' limitations may have been, as we cultivate the pro-creative power within our body's center, we can mother ourselves in the ways we need. We can know ourselves as the earth's daughters. We can know ourselves as beloved daughters of the Great Mother, the Mother of the Universe. We can know ourselves to be full, loved, enough.

Eating Disorders

What are eating disorders? They're clinically defined as mental and emotional illnesses that include anorexia nervosa, or self-starvation; binge eating, also called compulsive overeating; bulimia nervosa, binge eating that alternates with purging (vomiting or defecating induced by the abuse of laxatives); and "eating disorders not otherwise specified."[4]

The statistics are sobering. As reported by the National Eating Disorders Association, an estimated twenty-five million American girls and women are struggling with anorexia, bulimia, and binge eating.

Eating disorders are on the rise among women in midlife and beyond. One treatment center reports that nearly one-quarter of their residential patients are women thirty-five years of age and older. On average, these women who have been diagnosed with eating disorders in midlife have struggled with food and body image issues since they were teenagers, typically since they were fifteen years old.

Eating disorders can be fatal. The American Psychiatric Association's "Practice Guidelines for Eating Disorders" estimates that the death rate for eating disorders ranges from 5 to 20 percent. Anorexia is a leading cause of death among young women. Five to ten percent of anorexics die within ten years of the eating disorder's onset due to related causes, including cardiac arrest and suicide.

Eating disorders can follow from and in turn aggravate physiological factors that set a woman up for constant food cravings and stubborn weight gain. These factors can include imbalances in carbohydrate metabolism that manifest, for example, as hypoglycemia (low blood sugar) or insulin resistance; food allergies; and reactions to parasites and other natural and industrial pathogens.

Also, eating disorders can reflect personal, family, and cultural pressures to be thin, fit in, and maintain self-control. Research suggests that 80 percent of American women are dissatisfied with their appearance. At this very moment, one out of every two American women is on a diet; four out of five girls will be dieting by the time they're ten. Dieting drastically increases a teen girl's chance of developing an eating disorder. Among all ages, 8 out of every 100 people who diet will develop eating disorders.[5]

Dieting keeps us sorting food into categories of "good" and "bad." When we diet, we deny ourselves the possibility of listening to and acting upon our internal cues for when, what, and how much to eat and when we've had enough. We abandon our capacity to know, feed, and fulfill our own hungers. We keep following someone else's rules for how to feed ourselves; we keep looking in the mirror to see whether we're good enough yet. What else could we be doing with our time, energy, and attention? Something is out of order indeed.

Disordered eating has become the norm as much as dieting has. With so many girls and women encoding our distress in terms of food and the act of feeding ourselves, the term *eating disorder* may be losing its meaning. Maybe our unruly relationships with food display the pain of living in a culture that rules against women's self-respect. Maybe they signal our deep desire to live in a culture that affirms women and the pro-creative power we shelter within our bellies.

WHAT IS YOUR RELATIONSHIP TO FOOD?

Consider these questions:

- How do you know when you're hungry? How do you know when you've had enough to eat?

- How do you choose what you'll eat?

- What words do you use to rate different foods? For example, are some foods "safe"? Are other foods "forbidden"?

- How do you feel about yourself after you've eaten?

- How do you feel about eating when you're around other people?

- Do you ever binge in secret?

- Do you ever feel out of control when you are eating?

- How frequently do you weigh yourself?

- How often do you exercise because you think you have to burn off calories?

- In what situations do you eat when you're hungry and stop when you're satisfied?

- How many times a day do you think about food, weight, or dieting?

- How often do you diet?

The National Eating Disorders Association (NEDA) suggests that questions such as these can help identify a pattern of disordered eating.[6] For more information about eating disorders and disordered eating, contact NEDA's toll-free helpline at 800-931-2237.

PRIZE YOUR POWERHOUSE:
THE ENERGETIC DIMENSION

What is a living body? What makes it different from a machine? Life force. In Chinese, the word for "life force" is *qi* (pronounced "chee"). In Sanskrit, the language of yoga, it's *prana*. In Latin, *spiritus*. Women and men around the world have given their own names to the vital energy that animates life, that *is* life. Such names often associate this vital energy with the breath.

LIFE FORCE AROUND THE GLOBE

Women and men throughout the world name the vital energy that enlivens us.[7]

Arabic	*nafas*
Chinese	*qi*
Greek	*pneuma*
Hawaiian	*mana*
Hebrew	*ruah*
Iroquois	*orenda*
Japanese	*ki*
Lakotan	*wakan*
Latin	*anima, spiritus*
Sanskrit	*prana*

For millennia, many cultures have incorporated this energetic understanding of the body into their healing arts. The Asian practice of acupuncture, for example, maps the flow of the life force through the body. Treatments restore and promote health by relieving congestion, moderating excesses and deficiencies, and stimulating the life force to flow fully and freely.

Because life energy is an attribute of live bodies, energetic "structures" aren't necessarily found by dissecting cadavers in an anatomy lab. Consequently, different traditions name, locate, and describe them differently. Given all this variety, I offer you some names and descriptions derived from some of these traditions.

In this perspective, your body is a matrix for the flow of life energy. It's a power grid, a network of connecting currents of electricity. These currents conduct life force into every part of your body.

What moves this life force through your body? Where's the generator? It's in your belly. Your belly is the powerhouse that hosts the generator at the network's center.

The Power Source

The Japanese use a single word, *hara*, to name the belly both as a physical region of your body and as your connection to Source Energy. Your *hara* extends from the base of your ribs to the upper margin of your pubic bone, deepening inward to your spine. Within this region, a few inches below your navel, is your belly center — *tanden* in Japanese, *dantian* (pronounced "don-tee-en") in Chinese. To revisit this pivotal point, review Locating Your Center in chapter 1.

The Chinese name for this point, *dantian*, literally translates as "cinnabar field." Cinnabar, *dan*, is the metal that the ancient Chinese alchemists chose to transmute into the elixir of immortality. *Tian* denotes a field cultivated to produce food. *Dantian* implies that the belly is a field to be cultivated, a field that provides nourishment vital to life. An ancient Chinese name for this point translates as "Gate of the Mysterious Female."

Your belly stores the life force you were born with. It also receives and accumulates the additional life force you take in from food and water and through the breath. Your belly concentrates this life force and makes it available for distribution throughout your body. When you enliven your belly with movement, breath, and awareness, you're recharging the central power source that vitalizes your life.

The Power Grid

How does life energy move from your *hara* to the rest of your body? What's the distribution system? Here's a brief overview.

The Asian healing traditions consider the *hara* to be the center of a network of energy pathways called meridians. You receive, concentrate, and store the life force, the *qi*, within your *hara*, and these meridians conduct the *qi* throughout your body.

The network of meridians includes ten pathways, each named for and associated with an organ system. Occurring in pairs, these ten meridians are named Lung and Large Intestine, Spleen/Pancreas and Stomach, Heart and Small Intestine, Bladder and Kidney, and Liver and Gallbladder.

Two additional pathways are the Triple Heater and Heart Guardian meridians. As *qi* enters your body, the Triple Heater conducts the life force to your *hara*, where the vital energy accumulates and concentrates. The Triple Heater also conducts *qi* from your *hara* to each of the ten organ meridians, which in turn carry *qi* throughout your body. The Heart Guardian connects your *hara* with your heart.

In the tradition of yoga, the counterpart to the *hara* is the *kanda*, envisioned as a golden sphere or oval. As you breathe, the life force, *prana*, flows into your body and charges your *kanda*. Fourteen major energy channels called *nadis* arise from your *kanda* and branch into smaller pathways, distributing *prana* from your *kanda* through your entire body. Of the fourteen principal *nadis*, four of the most significant are *Saraswati, Sushumna, Ida,* and *Pingala.*

◈ The *Saraswati nadi* rises through the core of your body from your *kanda* to your tongue. It links

your belly with your capacity for speech, your
ability to speak your gut feelings.

◉ The *Sushumna nadi* rises from your *kanda* straight
up through the core of your body to the crown of
your head.

◉ The *Ida* and *Pingala nadis* rise from your *kanda* on
either side of the *Sushumna nadi*, spiraling around
the *Sushumna nadi* in a double helix. The *Ida* and
Pingala nadis conduct *prana* from the breath
into the *kanda*.

Where the *Ida* and *Pingala nadis* cross over the *Sushumna
nadi*, they give rise to the chakras, spinning wheels of energy.
Of the seven major chakras arranged along your body's vertical
axis, three are located within the region of your belly: the first
chakra, *Muladhara chakra*, at the base of your spine; the second chakra, *Swadhisthana chakra*, at the level of your uterus;
and the third chakra, *Manipura chakra*, at the center of your torso
beneath the lower border of your ribs.

The second chakra is sometimes confused with the *hara* (or
kanda) because its physical location seems to be the same. Energetically, though, the *hara* is at a level deeper than the second chakra.

Here's a way to explain their relationship: Picture your body
as a house. The *hara* is the furnace, the heat source, that's in the
basement. Heat travels from the central furnace through the ducts
that open into the vents installed in each room on the floor above.
The kitchen might be located on the floor right above the furnace
in the basement. But the vent that seems to be the source of heat

coming into the kitchen is just that, a vent; the heat source is the furnace in the basement below. Similarly, the *kanda* is the source of energy that activates the chakras, including the second chakra, through the *nadis*.

Hara is the Japanese word for both the belly and its soul power. Several Japanese phrases incorporate the word, pointing to its many levels of meaning. Here are some examples:[8]		
Japanese phrase	**Literal translation into English**	**Meaning in English**
Hara no okii hito	the one who has finished his belly	the fully mature person
Haratsuzumi wo utsu	to beat the belly drum	to lead a contented life
Haragei	belly art	any activity accomplished perfectly yet without effort
Hara de kangaenasai	please think with your belly	tap into your essential wisdom
Hara-goe	belly voice	a voice that expresses integrity and presence
Hara no naka wo watte misemasu	a person who shows what is inside his belly	one who speaks with genuine sincerity
Hara ga oki	a grand belly	a person who is understanding, compassionate, generous
Hara ga kirei	a clean belly	an honest person, one who has a clear conscience

THE BELLY'S SACRED POWER: A CROSS-CULTURAL REVIEW

- Among the !Kung tribe in Africa, the belly is known to contain the *n/um*, or "healing medicine," the vital life force that shamans stir and heat up with vigorous, ecstatic dancing. This life force boils up from the belly and the base of the spine, moving throughout the dancer's body. The energy is then available for healing others in the community.[9]

- The Sudanese understand the life force, *semangat*, to be focused within the navel; from that point it permeates the entire body.[10]

- In Indian and Tibetan traditions of yoga, the serpentine life force called *kundalini* lies coiled in the belly-centered *kanda*. Three major energy pathways, or *nadis* — the *Sushumna, Ida,* and *Pingala nadis* — rise from this source, spiraling upward through the body and generating the spinning wheels of energy known as chakras.

- Aboriginal Australians, too, have cultivated the serpent power dwelling within the body's center. As Robert Lawlor writes in *Voices of the First Day: Awakening in the Aboriginal Dreamtime,*

  [T]he Aboriginal tradition probably predated those of India and Tibet by 50,000 or 60,000 years. Long before such ideas existed in India, the Aboriginal men of high degree had consciously concentrated on the same body center (four fingers below the navel), where they said the cord of the great Rainbow Serpent (kundalini) lay coiled.... The Aborigines spoke of projecting psychic powers from these centers that were unhindered by time or space — powers that could bring healing life, death, and knowledge, or transfer thoughts.[11]

The body's center is revered in Native American traditions. In *Book of the Hopi*, for example, Frank Waters notes that the Hopi call it the "throne of the creator."[12] And Marilyn Youngbird, a tribal member of the Arikara and Hidatsa nations who lectures internationally on the Native Way, speaks of the importance of maintaining a spiritual, "umbilical" connection with the earth.[13] Similarly, Brooke Medicine Eagle says that "an umbilical cord connects you from your center to Mother Earth." She relates the importance of the belly to Native American teachings, especially the teaching of Buffalo Woman:

The message that Buffalo Woman gives us is that we need to understand and teach the experience of oneness. The belly is literally the place where you can put into practice Buffalo Woman's law of oneness and good relationship with all things. If you do it from that center, it's not something you have to think about, it's something that's there, it's something that connects you in a feeling way with all things around you.

That center, that belly-place in us is the place where the Great Mystery lives within us as two-leggeds. That's where creation literally takes place.

And it's not just children that we can create out of
that center of ourselves. When we receive vision,
when we fill ourselves with vision, we give birth to
those visions and make them real in the world out
of that place. All of our creation and our aliveness
can come out of that.[14]

◈ In Asia, Africa, and Europe, practitioners of alchemy
aspired to match the potency of a woman's womb. (Although alchemy became the basis for the science of
chemistry, it originated as a spiritual practice. By transforming matter in the external world, alchemists in-
tended to achieve an internal, personal transformation as
well.) The alchemists were seeking an elixir of immortality, a substance that would bestow healing, youthful-
ness, and life beyond death. They attempted to replicate
women's pro-creative power, the self-generating source
of life, in the crucible that symbolized a woman's belly.[15]

◈ In the Sufi tradition, the mystical expression of Islam,
kath refers to the belly's role in spiritual practice. The
whirling and spinning of Sufi dances concentrates awareness within the body's center, opening the way to union
with the divine.

◈ In Arabic, *rahim*, and in Hebrew, the same word in its
plural form, *rahamim*, each name the supreme Power of
Being and its quality of compassion. The root of *rahim*
is the Semitic *rhm*, meaning "womb," "loving-kindness,"
"mercy," and "nourishing tenderness."[16]

Meridians and the Body-Mind Connection

The Asian healing arts relate the five meridian pairs and their associated organs to five elemental forces of nature — metal, earth, fire, water, and wood — as well as to colors, tastes, smells, seasons, directions, dreams, mental capacities, emotions, actions, and functions. Through these correspondences, they detail the body-mind relationship and much more.

The table on the next page shows the functions and actions associated with each organ meridian.[17] These functions and actions apply to the related organ's way of being in the body, and also to a person's way of being in her life. If the Large Intestine meridian is congested, for example, a woman might be experiencing constipation, reluctance to let go and accept a loss, or difficulty in expressing grief.

Replenished by the *qi* you absorb from the food you eat, the water you drink, and the air you breathe, your *hara* is the source of the life energy that flows through the network of your meridians. When you enliven your *hara* with awareness, movement, and breath, life force can flow abundantly, restoring your body, mind, and emotions. Through its fundamental relationship to your network of meridians, your *hara* shapes your physical health and your mental and emotional well-being.

Chakras and the Body-Mind Connection

The seven major chakras, the spinning wheels of energy arranged along the body's vertical axis, each correspond to an aspect of awareness. If a chakra is spinning slowly, certain issues typically

Meridian pair	Element	Mental capacity	Emotion	Action	Function
Lung and large intestine	metal	sensitivity	courage, grief	establishing rhythmic order, releasing	stability
Spleen/ Pancreas and Stomach	earth	spontaneity	sympathy, worry	imagining, assimilating	integration
Heart and Small Intestine	fire	intuition	joy, impatience	commanding to action, sorting	excitement
Kidney and Bladder	water	ambition	gentleness, fear	creating, vitalizing	determination
Liver and Gallbladder	wood	clarity	kindness, anger	planning, decision making	control

arise in body and mind. Energizing the chakra enhances its related capacity for awareness and contributes to resolving the situation that's been problematic.

As the meridians do, the chakras give us a way to understand the body-mind relationships taking place in the belly and in the body as a whole. For example, emotional distress during childhood may damage the development of a woman's third chakra, associated with the intestines. Her symptoms of intestinal distress — such as abdominal pain and bloating, constipation, and diarrhea — may find healing as she strengthens her third chakra and resolves corresponding issues related to self-confidence and self-assertion.

The table that follows shows the concerns generally associated with each of the chakras.[18]

Chakra	Location	Related organs	Issue	Quality
Muladhara	base of spine	spine, immune system	survival	vitality
Swadhisthana	lower abdomen	pelvis, uterus, ovaries	sensuality	pleasure
Manipura	upper abdomen	intestines, liver, stomach	personal power	confidence
Anahata	heart	heart, lungs	intimacy	compassion
Vissudha	throat	throat, mouth	communication	creative expression
Ajna	forehead	brain, sense organs	perception	intuition
Sahasrara	crown	electromagnetic field	spiritual connection	sense of purpose

The *hara*-strengthening, *kanda*-boosting, belly-energizing exercises in part 2 activate your chakras. They enhance your capacity to express and enjoy the qualities related to each chakra.

These qualities — vitality, pleasure, confidence, compassion, creative expression, intuition, and sense of purpose — are attributes of soulful living as well. Developing and directing your *hara* power — the pro-creative power dwelling in your body's center, your soul power — brings these qualities to life.

You'll experience your connection with Source Energy yourself, in your own way, as you practice these exercises. Words have a limited ability to convey the experience. To give you a glimmer, I'll do what I can to describe my own experience.

MY EXPERIENCE OF *HARA*

When my belly feels active and alive, I feel warmth radiating from my belly's center. Sometimes I feel a pulsing in my belly; sometimes I feel a stirring sensation, as if a small world is spinning there. Often I feel a spaciousness and satisfaction in my belly, a sensation of being full and whole.

When my belly is energized, I feel settled and content, yet also ready for adventure. I feel that I belong to the world as a whole. I'm living in the center of my world, and I feel at home wherever I go. I experience a resonance between my body and the earth's body, a linking vibration, a mutual attraction.

MATRIX ME

I am
the mother planet's
  life process.

As I plant my feet
anywhere upon her surface,

my belly center resonates
with my earth mother's middle.

She rises up through me,
our geologies join.

This earth world's center,
     be it her belly,
then my belly
     is her heart,
my heart,
     her knowing eye.

She is alive to the heat of my feeling.
She is alive to the light of my seeing.

I am alive to the words of this mother world.
I am alive to the worlds of this mother's word.

I rest in her.
The ground comes up to matrix me
And I am resting in her.

WHAT'S SO GOOD ABOUT YOUR BELLY?

Your belly — physically, emotionally, and energetically — is the center of your life. Your belly contains the vital organs that orchestrate your digestion, respiration, reproduction, immunity, and more. Your belly is a wealth of emotional intelligence, keeping the code for naming your core issues and reclaiming your procreative power. Your belly is a cauldron of life energy, storing *qi* and sending it through your entire body.

What is the thread running through these three dimensions? The breath.

Breathe, and you supply your body and brain with oxygen. Breathe, and you allow yourself to feel. Breathe, and you recharge your *hara* with vital energy.

How do you breathe fully and deeply? You let your belly move freely with the tide of your breath. As in the exercise that follows, you breathe in a way that fills your body with an ocean of energy.

FULL-BODY BREATHING

1. Sit or stand comfortably, or lie on your back with a pillow under your knees to ease your lower back.

2. Rest your palms on your lower abdomen, placing the center of your hands over your belly's center. Deepen your awareness into this point. What do you feel here?

3. Enter into the Centering Breath. As you inhale, see and feel the breath activating this center point, expanding from here to fill the entire volume of your body — all the way to your fingertips and toes, all the way up to your scalp and down to your perineum — with light, warmth, and energy.

4. As you exhale, see and feel the breath returning to concentrate at your center point, making it even livelier, stronger, brighter.

5. Stay with this image and sense of breathing for ten or more cycles of breath. What do you notice? How do you feel in body and mind?

6. Gradually return your attention to the present moment.

BECOMING *HARA*-FIED

Now you have an idea of what's rumbling around in your belly. You've become acquainted with some of the physical, emotional, and energetic aspects of being in your body's center. You've got vocabulary, you've got concepts, you've got language for talking about the nature of *hara* and the benefits of firing up your *hara* power, your power to promote creation.

Let's move into the realm of direct experience. Part 2 invites you to dip into the wisdom and power your belly shelters. How? By enlivening your body's center with compassionate awareness and invigorating movement and breath.

Developing and directing your *hara* power, the pro-creative power dwelling in your body's center, is a continuing process of discovery. As a friend once reminded me, *hara* is the ocean. As deep as you go, you can always go deeper. Welcome to the adventure of a lifetime!

Part Two

Sparking Your *Soul* Power

Chapter Five

Practice Pointers

Now is the time to move from idea into action. Here you'll learn to use movement, breath, and body awareness to magnify your experience of soulful living.

SOUL QUALITIES

Vitality, pleasure, confidence, compassion, creativity, intuition, purpose — these are seven qualities of the soul made manifest. They're seven attributes of living a gutsy life, seven expressions of your soul power. In this part of the book, you'll have the opportunity to focus on each of these qualities in turn. What does *vitality* mean to you? What pleasures really please you? What's the difference between arrogance and confidence? How do you express and receive compassion? What are the rewards of expressing your creativity and trusting your intuition? How does a sense of purpose simplify and enrich your life?

You'll also have the opportunity to magnify each of these qualities by kindling the soul power that is their source. In each of the following chapters, in relation to each quality, you'll find the following:

- Two playful, provocative ways to deepen your appreciation of your belly. These awareness exercises encourage you to be creative and have fun in the process of befriending your belly.

- A breathing pattern that engages your imagination in guiding the life force concentrated in your belly throughout your body. Developing your ability to direct vital energy in this way enhances your capacity for self-healing.

- A belly-energizing move, adapted from the classic tradition of hatha yoga, from the *hara*-charging style of yoga developed by Masahiro Oki, or from another approach to movement as a healing art. These moves enable you to fire up the pro-creative power concentrated in your body's center.

- A drawing and description of an ancient artifact that expresses our ancestors' reverence for the Source Energy dwelling within women's bellies. These images convey aspects of our pro-creative power — our capacities for cycling, holding space, nourishing,

regenerating, expressing, connecting, and being
present — that are ours to affirm today as well. Let
these images invite you to renew and reinvent
humankind's tradition of honoring a woman's belly
as sacred, not shameful.

The seven soul qualities commingle, of course, building upon and reinforcing each other. Vitality increases your receptivity to pleasure; being receptive to pleasure enhances your confidence. Self-confidence equips you to feel compassion for, rather than envy of, others. Motivated by compassion, not the need for others' approval, you bypass performance anxiety and ease into creative expression. Expressing yourself freely gives you more access to your intuitive knowing; your intuition clarifies your sense of purpose.

Because the qualities relate to each other in this way, I suggest you explore them in the sequence in which I've presented them. Refer to the Guidelines for Practice later in this chapter. They will help you learn the belly-energizing moves easily and safely. In chapter 13, you'll find suggestions for designing a belly-energizing practice of your own and incorporating it into your life. Integrating The Gutsy Women's Workout as a regular feature in your life is a magnificent way to honor your body and yourself.

BEING GENTLE WITH YOURSELF

Remember that all of the exercises in this book are potentially transformative. They're all ways to ignite the spark of the Power of Being that's been entrusted to you. They're all opportunities to experience this power's capacity to provoke shifts in your body, mind, and emotions.

Accordingly, your first priority is to be gentle with yourself. Go slowly. Don't push yourself. Consult your inner guidance — your central authority — and do just as much as you're ready for. There's no rush. Be gradual in exploring new awareness exercises, new breathing patterns, new belly-energizing moves. You don't have to prove anything. You're already enough.

Return frequently to the core principles and core practices: Giving Yourself Room to Breathe, Locating Your Center, Centering the Breath, Naming Your Feelings, and Setting Your Intention. These practices and their corresponding principles will help ground and anchor you in the present.

If you begin to feel some distress, simply do less. Or give it all a rest for a few days and begin again when you feel ready. You might take time out to review the cultural exposé in chapter 2. You might also take a look at the gruesome details of our culture's assault on women's bellies in appendix 1. You'll understand the courage we demonstrate as we reclaim our pro-creative power. You'll understand the compassion we deserve as we deepen our awareness into our bellies. And you'll likely find a context for whatever discomfort you may be experiencing, making your feelings more manageable. If your discomfort continues, be sure to obtain the professional assistance that will address your individual needs.

THE LEARNING PROCESS

As you learn each move, you'll progress through a series of stages. For the most fun — and to avoid confusing or overwhelming yourself — learn and practice one move thoroughly before going on to the next. Here are some pointers for organizing your learning process:

1. Begin by focusing on the physical details of the exercise — what to do with your arms and hands, where to place your feet, when to bend your knees, where to direct your gaze.

2. Then attend to how you're coordinating the movement with the breath — either the Centering Breath or the Energizing Breath, depending on the particular exercise. Notice which phase of the movement accompanies the inhalation and which phase of the movement accompanies the exhalation.

3. At first, practice just a few repetitions of each move. As you're ready, increase your repetitions to the number suggested for each exercise.

4. Once you're comfortable with the details of the movement and the ways in which your breath animates your body, you'll be ready to comprehend the move as a complete gesture, rather than as a sequence of things to do. At this point, experiment with generating the movement from your belly and with your breath. What does it mean to let your *hara* power be the source of all the action taking place through your torso, legs, arms, neck, and head? How is your whole body, out to your

fingertips, down to your toes, and all the way to the roots of your hair, expressing the dynamism of your body's center?

5. As you're ready, add another refinement: imbue your movement with — literally incorporate — an image, informing your action with meaning and intention. The instructions for each move suggest a corresponding image. You might move through chapter 6's Bright Blessings, for example, with the image and intention that you're gathering blessings from the earth, trees, and sky, and storing these blessings in your body's center. Experiment and see what other images emerge for you.

Each gesture offers many layers of meaning, waiting for you to experience and name them in ways that are uniquely yours. The possibilities are endless. As a move becomes truly your own gesture, you may find that it also becomes an affirmation, or a prayer. Express your experience as you're inspired — in words, music, colors, and form. Poems, songs, chants, stories, paintings, and sculptures are waiting in the wings!

GUIDELINES FOR PRACTICE

Each of the next seven chapters presents a belly-energizing exercise. I've selected the exercises from the original series of twenty-three moves that I have shared with women and practiced daily myself for more than a decade. Together, these seven exercises form a well-balanced, invigorating sequence that you can easily practice in five to seven minutes.

Of these seven moves, three (Belly Bowl, Tree, and Alignment) employ the Centering Breath, which you've already encountered as a core practice. The other four moves (Bright Blessings, Power Centering, Lily, and Wings) employ the more vigorous Energizing Breath. You'll find instructions for the Energizing Breath later in this chapter.

Begin each session of learning and practicing the moves by limbering your body with the three warm-up/warm-down exercises you'll find in this chapter: the Side Stretches, Diagonal Stretches, and Cradle. These exercises prepare your body to do the more vigorous moves with safety and pleasure. End your session with these same three exercises to smooth your transition into the rest of your day's activities.

> Looking back on how I've practiced, I can identify four stages. First, I learned the movements and how to make time in my life for doing them. This was kind of a mental process. The second stage was when I could do the exercises comfortably, being in my body without having to think about how to do the movements. The third stage was being conscious of the energy, how I could direct the energy I was generating. The fourth stage was healing, when the movements gave me insights into the problems I was facing.
>
> — Susan

To receive the benefits of these belly-energizing exercises, you don't have to make any heroic effort. There's no need to strain. Your body learns best when the experience is easy and pleasurable.

You don't have to go to extremes. These moves are not about struggling to match some external ideal. They're about coming home to yourself. They're about the pleasures of returning to your center.

If you were attending a workshop, I'd be teaching you the belly-energizing moves with enthusiasm and delight. I'd also have my eagle eye out for your comfort and safety. Since I'm not with you at the moment, read and abide by the following preparations and the do's and don'ts. Use them to ensure that your practice is safe, comfortable, and rewarding. If you are pregnant, be sure to read the section "If You Are Pregnant" on page 138.

Remember, there's no need to strain. The beginning and end of this practice are the same: loving your belly, your body, and yourself.

Preparations

- Practice on an empty stomach. Allow one hour for digestion following a light meal and at least two hours following a full meal.

- Give yourself ample time, free from interruption.

- Wear comfortable clothes — with a loose waistband, of course. Remove your glasses, jewelry, and dangling earrings to avoid injury. Practice in bare feet on a nonslip surface, or wear gym shoes with flat, relatively thin soles.

- Create a pleasant, well-ventilated, comfortably warm environment for yourself. Post the image of your intention that you created in chapter 1 (or have since revised) on the wall in front of you, placing it at eye level to use as your visual focus during your practice.

@ Keep a journal, blank paper, and markers handy if you'd like to follow your movement practice with an awareness exercise such as Dialogue with Your Inner Wisdom (page 202) or Draw Out Your Deepest Knowing (page 214).

As You Begin

Start with the core practices detailed in chapter 1 and:

@ Give yourself room to breathe

@ Locate your center

@ Enter into the Centering Breath

@ Name your feelings in this moment

@ Set your intention

Then move on to the following:

@ Prepare for vigorous movement with the three warm-up/warm-down exercises.

@ Move slowly and smoothly. Attend to what you're doing.

- Move within your comfort zone; never strain, push, or force yourself. As detailed below, do not overdo practicing the exercises.

- Ease out of vigorous movement with the three warm-up/warm-down exercises.

Do

- As with any new exercise program, consult with your health care provider in advance to determine whether and how these breathing and movement exercises are suitable for you. Ask for specific guidance to address your individual needs, especially if you are pregnant or have a history of any of the following:

  - Back, shoulder, hip, or knee injury or pain
  - Abdominal injury or pain
  - Uncontrolled high blood pressure
  - Asthma, diabetes, hypoglycemia, kidney disease
  - Heart disease, cancer, or risk for stroke
  - Prolapsed uterus or bladder

- During menstruation, adjust your practice according to what's appropriate for you. You may, for example, prefer to practice the moves very gently and slowly during the first day of your menstrual flow.

Do Not

◉ Do not overdo the exercises, particularly the more vigorous movement and breathing patterns. Here's why: The Energizing Breath adds oxygen to the body and brain. That's good. Still, when beginning to practice the Energizing Breath (either alone or in combination with Bright Blessings, Power Centering, Lily, and Wings), some people may feel slightly light-headed or dizzy with oxygen in unusually abundant supply. If that's the case for you, at first do only a few repetitions of the exercise, and do them slowly. Pay particular attention to the sensation of energy moving from your belly and streaming down through your legs, through your feet, into the ground, and into the earth below. Over time, and as you're ready, gradually increase your practice to the number of repetitions suggested for each exercise. With practice, you'll increase your capacity to absorb abundant oxygen with comfort and ease.

◉ Do not chew gum and attempt to do the exercises at the same time. Really!

IF YOU ARE PREGNANT

If you are pregnant, you may still be able to do many of the exercises. Be sure to follow these recommendations:

Do

- Discuss with your health care provider whether and how this program might be appropriate for you, given the progress of your pregnancy and your own health status. The Perineal Squeeze in chapter 3, for example, may be particularly useful in helping you strengthen your pelvic floor. Ask for specific guidance in selecting and modifying this and other exercises to suit your individual needs.

- Practice only the Centering Breath and other breathing patterns that don't require a vigorous abdominal contraction with the exhalation.

- Practice Bright Blessings, Power Centering, Lily, and Wings with the Centering Breath, rather than with the Energizing Breath.

- When practicing Wings, keep your feet in place to avoid losing your balance. For the same reason, keep your heels on the floor when practicing Tree.

Do Not

- Do not forcefully compress your belly while exhaling.
- Do not hold your breath for an extended period of time.

WARM-UP/WARM-DOWN EXERCISES

Use these three exercises to prepare your body for movement and also to bring your practice session to a close. Feel free to do more repetitions than the number I've suggested to ensure you've limbered up thoroughly.

SIDE STRETCHES

Repeat three times, with the Centering Breath.

1. Stand with your feet wider than your hips. Point your toes out about forty-five degrees. Bend your knees slightly, keeping them directly over your toes. Bring your arms overhead.

2. With your left hand, clasp your right wrist. Sink down, bending your knees further for a moment. Then slowly lengthen and stretch your whole right side, pressing from your waist down through your right foot and reaching up from your waist through your right wrist and fingertips. Gently roll your right shoulder back, opening it and allowing your right arm to stretch above, rather than in front of, your head. Explore this stretch for three to five breaths.

3. Slowly return to center. Release your right wrist. Notice and feel what's happening in your body. Compare the sensations in your right and left sides.

4. Now, to balance left and right, with your right hand clasp your left wrist. Sink down, bending your knees further for a moment. Then slowly lengthen and stretch your whole

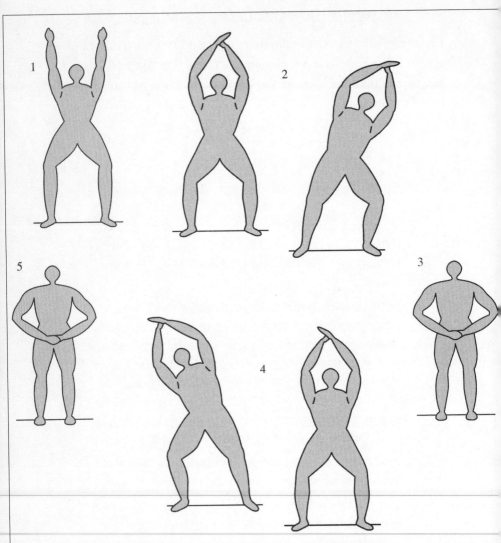

Side Stretches

left side, pressing from your waist down through your left foot and reaching up from your waist through your left wrist and fingertips. Gently roll your left shoulder back, opening it and allowing your left arm to stretch above, rather than in front of, your head. Explore this stretch for three to five breaths.

5. Slowly return to center. Release your left wrist. Notice and feel what's happening in your body. Compare the sensations in your left and right sides.

As you move through the Side Stretches, investigate what it means to invite, rather than force, your body to open. As you become familiar with these stretches, notice how — by defining your body's left and right borders — you're also calling attention to the spaciousness within these borders, your body's core.

DIAGONAL STRETCHES

Repeat three times, with the Centering Breath.

1. Stand with your feet parallel, hip-width apart. Bend your knees slightly, keeping them directly over your toes. Rest your palms lightly on your belly, over your body's center.

2. Lift your palms a few inches away from your body and roll your hands one over the other in front of your belly, stirring up the cauldron of vital energy in your body's center.

3. Shift your weight to the right, into your right foot and leg. Now bend and lift your left leg and take a wide step to your

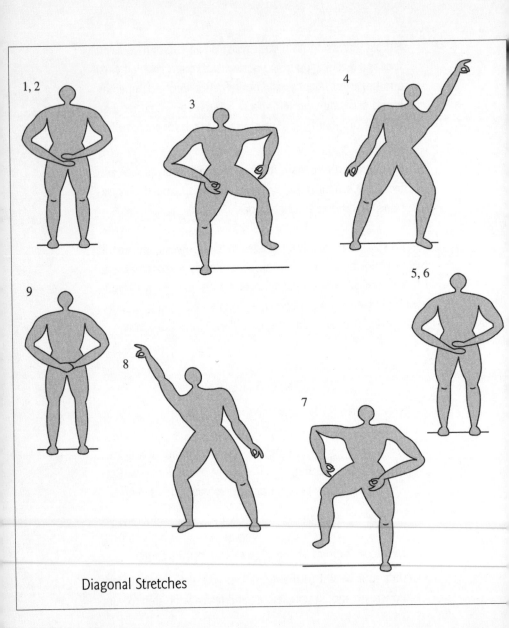

Diagonal Stretches

left, placing your foot on the ground so that your left toes point out about forty-five degrees. (Your right foot remains in place, toes pointing straight forward.) Bending your left knee directly over your toes, lean into your left foot and leg. At the same time, press your right foot and leg into the ground, keeping your right knee still slightly bent.

4. As you're stepping to the left, create a circle with the thumb and first finger of each hand and stretch your left arm up past your left ear, stretching your right arm down toward the ground along the same diagonal. Extend from your body's center up through your left arm and hand and at the same time down through your right foot, arm, and hand. Explore this stretch for three to five breaths.

5. Shift your weight toward center and return your left foot and leg to the hip-width stance. Roll your hands one over the other in front of your belly, then rest your palms over your body's center. Notice and feel what's happening in your body. Compare the sensations in your right and left sides.

6. Now, to balance left and right, once again lift your palms and roll your hands one over the other in front of your belly.

7. Shift your weight to the left, into your left foot and leg. Now bend and lift your right leg and take a wide step to your right, placing your foot on the ground so that your right toes point out about forty-five degrees. (Your left foot remains in place, toes pointing straight forward.) Bending your right knee directly over your toes, lean into your right foot and leg. At the same time, press your left foot and leg into the ground, keeping your left knee slightly bent.

8. As you're stepping to the right, create a circle with the thumb and first finger of each hand and stretch your right arm up past your right ear, stretching your left arm down toward the ground along the same diagonal. Extend from your body's center up through your right arm and hand and at the same time down through your left foot, arm, and hand. Explore this stretch for three to five breaths.

9. Shift your weight toward center and return your right foot and leg to the hip-width stance. Roll your hands one over the other in front of your belly, then rest your palms over your body's center. Notice and feel what's happening in your body. Compare the sensations in your left and right sides.

As you become familiar with these stretches, feel how the diagonals run through your body and your belly, and note the point at which they intersect.

CRADLE

Repeat five times, with the Centering Breath.

1. Stand with your feet wider than your hips. Point your toes out about forty-five degrees. Bend your knees slightly, keeping them directly over your toes.

2. Let your arms be loose and your neck and shoulders be soft. Bending your knees a bit more, alternate pressing one hip forward and then the other, generating a gentle rocking motion around the central axis of your spine.

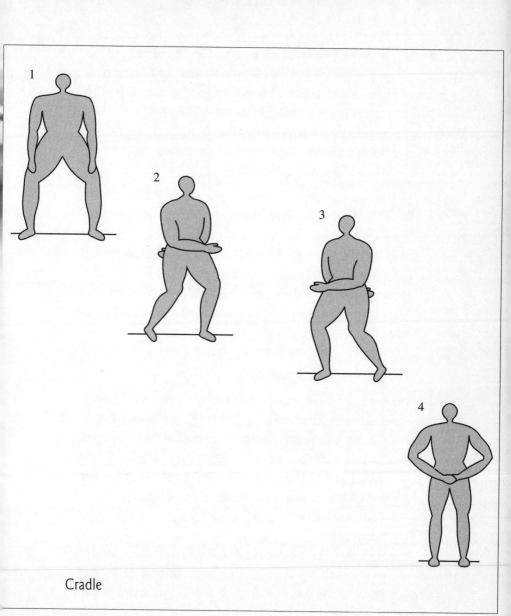

Cradle

3. Experiment with expanding the motion of your pelvis so that your spine enjoys a gentle twist as your arms swing easily from side to side, even beginning to wrap around your rib cage. Allow your heels to alternate in lifting from the ground to facilitate the spinal twist. (For example, your right heel lifts as your torso, neck, and head are turning to the left.)

4. Notice and feel what's happening in your body. In the same way you'd cherish a newborn nestled in your arms, cherish the life force your belly cradles.

Greek words for "cradle" and "cradling," such as *baubauein*, *baubalidsein*, and *bakale*, echo the name of Baubo, the belly goddess. Even in modern times, *baubalidsa* is an affectionate Greek name for a child, one who is cradled in sheltering care.

ENERGIZING BREATH

The Energizing Breath, incorporated in Bright Blessings (chapter 6), Power Centering (chapter 8), Lily (chapter 9), and Wings (chapter 10), calls for breathing in through your nose and breathing out through your wide-open mouth — let your jaw hang open! Your belly serves as a bellows, expanding to draw the breath in and pulling back toward your spine to press the breath out.

Preparation:

1. Standing or sitting comfortably, place one palm in front of your mouth. Place your other palm on your belly, your thumb at the level of your navel, your fingers resting below.

2. Have you ever fogged a mirror with your breath as you're getting ready to clean it? Breathe out into your upraised hand two or three times as if you were fogging a mirror. At the same time, notice how the hand that's on your belly is moving. Most likely, it moves in toward your spine as your belly contracts with each exhalation.

3. You might notice a sound emerging as you exhale. It's simply the sound of the breath passing through your throat and out your mouth. Don't strain your throat. You don't have to use your vocal chords or any of the muscles in your throat to expel the breath; you don't have to force the exhalation. Your belly takes charge of sending out the breath.

Practice:

1. Sit or stand comfortably. Place your hands lightly on your lower abdomen.

2. Keeping your mouth closed, expand your belly to draw the breath in through your nose.

3. Gently yet firmly pull your belly back in toward your spine, pressing the breath out as you open your mouth to allow the exhalation. Let your throat and shoulders remain completely relaxed.

4. Continue with two or three slow repetitions. As you become comfortable with the practice, gradually increase to five to seven repetitions.

What do you feel happening in your belly? How do you feel in body and mind?

Remember: If you feel dizzy or light-headed, start with only a few slow repetitions of the Energizing Breath. Attend to the current of energy moving from your belly and flowing down through your legs, through your feet, into the ground, and into the earth below. Then gradually increase the number of repetitions. With practice, you'll increase your capacity to comfortably absorb an abundant supply of oxygen.

Now you're ready to sample the pleasures of activating your body's center with the sequence of moves that follow. Enjoy!

Chapter Six

Vitality: Keep Looking and Feeling Great

"Now I know why you always look like you're in love." That's what one woman told me after moving through some of the belly-energizing exercises with me. She had some of the same sparkle herself. No matter what your body shape or size is, no matter what age you are, no matter what your bone structure might be, when your energy is strong and steady, you look and feel good. You're vivacious. You're vibrant. You're full of vitality.

Your belly is your powerhouse, your life-energy generator. As you've come to appreciate, your belly is vital to your physical well-being. Your abdominal organs transform your food into nourishment. Among a host of other favors, they also circulate your blood and boost your immunity. They keep you alive.

Your belly is central to your emotional health as well. Enabling you to breathe deeply, your belly is your best friend when it comes to helping you relax, release stress, and enjoy restful sleep.

The Dispense with Stress and Sleep Easy exercises enlist your body's center in dispelling tension. Breathing into Three Dimensions expands your belly breathing and revitalizes your whole body. Energizing your belly with Bright Blessings lifts your spirits and kindles the inner glow that becomes radiance for all to see.

TENSION-RELIEVING EXERCISES

In one way or another, stress is resistance to *what* is, the reality of the present moment. Whenever I'm fabricating hopes and fears about the future or wishing I could time-travel and change the past, I'm stressing big-time. I'm neglecting what's real and true right now. And I'm ignoring the blessings all around me, blessings that are mine if I'll notice and receive them with gratitude.

For the first time I experienced fully what it means to be in touch with my belly. Now I've manifested a power which has left me with a sense of appreciation for being a woman. My entire being — body, mind, and spirit — filled with a beauty sensed both inside and out. With each pulse I grew more beautiful. This sense of being rests with me. In connecting with my belly, I have found that I am part of a greater whole.

— *Giovanna*

Opening the way for a variety of physical and emotional ailments, constant stress drains your vitality. To banish stress and boost your vitality, focus your attention on your body's center and breathe in a way that calms your mind and soothes your frazzled nerves. As tension dissolves and stress subsides, you'll feel both relaxed and alert to the goodness that surrounds you.

DISPENSE WITH STRESS

This exercise draws on the inspiration of Seigen Yamaoka's *The Art and the Way of Hara.*[1] If you're pregnant, refer to the practice pointers in chapter 5 before beginning this exercise.

1. Sit or stand comfortably, or lie on your back with a pillow under your knees to ease your lower back.

2. Keeping your mouth closed, slowly inhale through your nose, expanding your belly to draw the breath in.

3. Having inhaled fully, now push your belly farther out to inhale even more.

4. Open your mouth and exhale slowly, allowing your belly to sink back toward your spine.

5. Having exhaled completely, now pull your belly farther in to exhale even more.

6. Repeat up to ten times. Notice how tension fades away.

In the absence of deep and restful sleep, the effects of stress accumulate. Sleep revitalizes and rejuvenates your body and mind. As you're sleeping, your body discharges toxins through the breath and skin. Your mind defines the dilemmas of your life through the color, form, and story of dreams. Your dreams, in fact, showcase your gut instincts. When we're asleep, we don't have the "presence of mind" to deny our deepest wisdom.

For me, an awareness of *hara* comes from carefully listening to and acting on my dreams.

— *Ann*

Insomnia is becoming epidemic. The number of prescriptions filled for sleeping pills totaled about forty-two million in 2005. One in ten Americans reports they frequently struggle to fall asleep or have difficulty sleeping through the night.[2]

Insomnia plays out a discouraging predicament: The restless mind prevents sleep, increasing fatigue. Fatigue aggravates mental tension, again preventing sleep.

We need to rest well, especially when we're anxious or feeling overwhelmed. Yet that's when sleep seems entirely out of reach. The mind is chattering away, the body is tense.

Thankfully, the body's center can serve as your doorway into sleep. As you focus your attention on your belly and your breathing, tension drains away from body and mind. Slumberland calls you across the threshold.

I tried the following practice for the first time during a spell of tossing restlessly around in my bed. I completed the five repetitions and grumbled, "Well, this doesn't seem to be working." The next thing I knew, it was morning, and I felt refreshed.

SLEEP EASY

This exercise adapts another technique Seigen Yamaoka describes in *The Art and the Way of Hara*.[3] Again, if you're pregnant, refer to the practice pointers in chapter 5.

1. Lie on your back with your legs fully extended; place a pillow under your knees to ease your lower back.

2. Keeping your mouth closed, inhale slowly through your nose, expanding your belly to draw the breath in.

3. As you hold the breath in, contract your belly and pull it down toward your spine.

4. Holding the breath, tense the muscles in your legs, arms, face, chest, back, and buttocks, contracting every muscle from the outer edges of your body toward the center.

5. Now, still holding the breath in and keeping every muscle tight, push your belly out and hold it out for a slow count of five.

6. Open your mouth and exhale slowly. At the same time, totally relax all your muscles.

7. Repeat as many as five times. Notice how restlessness gives way to repose.

BREATHING INTO THREE DIMENSIONS

1. Sit comfortably. Allow your breath to sink down into your belly, and enter into the Centering Breath. Focus your awareness within you body's center.

2. Notice how both your belly and the area around the base of your spine move as your breath expands from and retracts toward your body's center. This front-to-back dimension is the dimension of depth. Experience the sensation of the breath moving through your body in this dimension.

3. Notice, too, how your ribs and the sides of your body move as your breath expands from and retracts toward your body's

center. This side-to-side dimension is the dimension of width. Experience the sensation of the breath moving through your body in this second dimension.

4. Notice how your spine moves as your breath expands from and retracts toward your body's center. This up-and-down dimension is the dimension of height. Experience the sensation of the breath moving through your body in this third dimension.

5. Closing your eyes, take a few moments to experience the images and sensations occurring as your breath moves through the three-dimensional volume of your body.

6. Gradually return your awareness to this time and place.

THE POWER OF CYCLING

A miniature shrine in ancient Greece displayed this figure whose hands point to her belly. Three parallel lines mark both the front and back of her torso. On her back, three more lines shape a triangle at the base of her spine.

Your power to promote creation is the power to cycle through time, space, and form. A cycle implies at least three phases or stages: beginning, middle, and end; waxing, full, and waning moon; maiden, mother, and crone. In folklore and fairy tales, it's the third sister or the third attempt that fulfills the promise: the third time's the charm.

When you allow cycles to take place in your life, you can receive the blessings each stage has to offer. If I'm anxiously trying

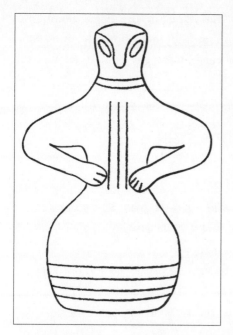

Tri-lines mark this figurine
found in a miniature shrine.
Thessaly, Greece, c. 5000 B.C.E.

to make my face and figure look like a teenager's when I'm past
fifty, I'm missing out on the wise-cracking self-assurance that
comes with aging gracefully. If I'm still trying to "suck it up" and
flatten my stomach, I'm missing out on the *hara* power that's all
the more accessible to me past menopause.

What are the cycles turning in your life? How do you accept
the blessings of each phase?

As you move through Bright Blessings, notice the three realms
you define as your arms move up to shoulder level, out to your
sides, and up overhead. See and feel yourself invoking the power of
cycling into your world and storing that power within your belly.

As one woman says, "Bright Blessings affirms that all life, all respect, everything begins and ends in the earth-womb, the mother-belly. I feel that within my belly, my womb, the universe is born. I receive the energy of earth, trees, sky — all come into my womb, to heal and be healed."

BRIGHT BLESSINGS

Repeat five times, with the Energizing Breath.

1. Stand with your feet parallel, hip-width apart. Bend your knees slightly, keeping them over your toes. Lengthen your arms alongside your body.

2. As you inhale, lift your arms up and forward to shoulder level.

3. Continue inhaling as you spread your arms out to the sides.

4. Still inhaling, lift your arms up overhead, overlapping your thumbs and fingertips to shape a triangle.

5. Exhaling, bend your knees further and bring your hands down to your body's center, pressing lightly into your belly. Notice and feel any images and sensations that are occurring in your body.

Breath and image: Applying the Energizing Breath, inhale as your arms reach forward, out, and up: you're gathering blessings from the earth, the trees, the sky. Exhale through your open mouth as your hands return to your belly: you're receiving these blessings and storing them in your body's center.

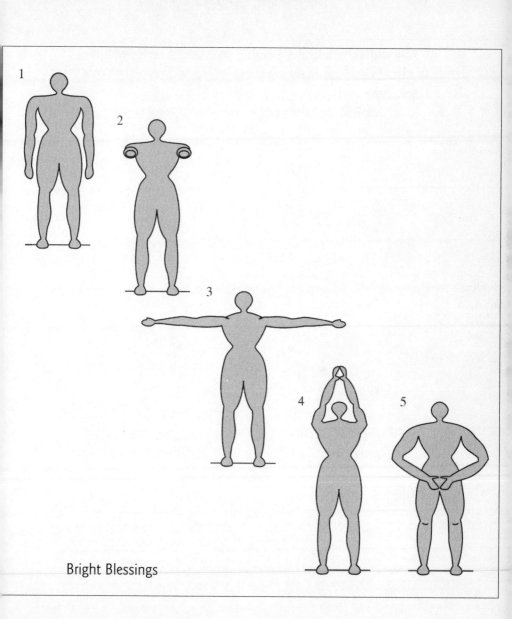

Bright Blessings

See and feel a bright line linking your body's center with the earth's center, anchoring you in a strong and supportive cord of connection.

Question for reflection: What blessings are you willing to receive from the earth, the trees, the sky?

Chapter Seven

Pleasure:
Spice Up Your Sensuality

"A majority of women prefer reading a good book to having sex." That may or may not be just an urban legend. But when I pose this possibility to friends, they nod with a knowing look. The National Health and Social Life Survey reveals that one in three American women between the ages of eighteen and fifty-nine lacks interest in sex for several months or more during the course of a year.[1]

With all the responsibilities of work, home, and family, many women are exhausted by the time they finally get to bed. Who has the energy for sex?

Despite the media hype that would make us believe that everyone except us is having glamorous sexual escapades in glorious abundance, merely seven out of one hundred American women have sex more than three times a week. Nearly two-thirds of American women engage in sex no more than a few times a month.[2]

What is sexual pleasure? It's the play of sexual energy, one expression of your life energy as a whole. When you have more energy, you experience more pleasure.

Sexual pleasure is also nature's way of interesting us in regenerating the human race, procreating in the literal sense. Our sexual urges play out our species' instinct for self-preservation as well as our own.

The sexual pleasure we enjoy as we kindle our soul power is one domain within the larger realm of sensual pleasure that opens up to us. As you cultivate your pro-creative power, you're all the more aware of the erotic energy that hums all around you. Romance, candlelight, and satin sheets are not required.

> I'm claiming my wholeness as a woman that I've never had before. Energizing my belly has enabled me to gain an openness and release of sensual, sexual energy and healing. I feel increased connectedness to the feminine.
>
> — Mimi

As you energize your body's center, you awaken to the life force that's tingling through your body and bursting through the world. Exhilaration is yours to find in the textured taste of an apple, a bird's morning chirp, the soft touch of water spilling through your fingers, the fragrance of fresh air, the cerulean blue sky.

The Decorate Your Underwear and Let Yourself Laugh exercises celebrate your body's center as a source of pleasure. With celebration comes freedom to express your sensuality and sexuality in ways that are engaging, fulfilling, and comfortable for you. Glowing

Globe adds color and image to intensify your experience of belly breathing. Mobilizing your hips with Belly Bowl prepares your body to take all the more delight in the pleasures of sense and sexuality.

PLEASURE-PROMOTING EXERCISES

Decorate your underwear with a belly-celebrating design and you'll be making a stunning fashion statement; you're proudly claiming your pro-creative, life-affirming power as your own.

You'll also be in good company. In the nineteenth century, Elizabeth Smith Miller designed roomy pantaloons to be worn under short skirts, freeing women from the confining fashions of the day. Her cousin, suffragist Amelia Jenks Bloomer, popularized the undergarments through her monthly newspaper, *The Lily*. Elizabeth Cady Stanton and others leading the struggle for women's rights made a point of wearing these Bloomers, as they came to be known. They put their Bloomers away, though, when the popular press focused on their underwear and neglected the more substantial issues of women's emancipation.

> I experienced a deep, deep orgasm — and it was heightened and elongated due to breathing deeply. I realized that I was doing this deep breathing naturally. Wow.
>
> — Tricia

You never know when your own undercover wardrobe will come in handy. One woman who stood with others in a weekly silent vigil for peace learned that the police would be challenging the group's right to assemble in a public place. She made sure to wear her "power panties" that day — just in case the police would be making arrests and doing strip searches.

DECORATE YOUR UNDERWEAR

1. Gather your supplies: fabric paints and glitter, paintbrushes, cotton underpants in your favorite color, a circular paper plate, and masking tape.

2. Insert the paper plate into the center of the underpants to separate front from back. Fold the side edges of the undies around to the back of the plate and fasten them with masking tape so the fabric won't move as you paint on the front.

3. Enter into the Centering Breath and consider the ways in which your belly serves you. Let the sense of gratitude fill you fully as you take paintbrush in hand and apply a design to the fabric. You might paint a symbol that has special meaning for you, or an image that has come to you in a dream.

    Continue until you've created a pair of undies that honors your belly in style.

What makes you laugh so hard your belly shakes?

My neighbor told me that last night her husband's Viagra got stuck in his throat. Nothing much happened, but this morning he woke up with a stiff neck.

I told this joke to some friends and we laughed. I laughed so hard my belly quaked. All the tension in my body broke up into tiny pieces and fell away.

What is a belly laugh? It's a tremor rippling through your

tissues, tickling your innards. It's an inner shimmy that makes the cells of your body dance with delight.

In the ancient Greek story of Demeter's search for her daughter Persephone, belly goddess Baubo saves the day with the bawdy joking that makes Demeter laugh. The laughter dispels Demeter's grief and allows her to continue looking for and eventually find her daughter. With Persephone's return, the earth's fertility returns as well.

If it's been too long since your last good guffaw, now's the time to get the laughter going again.

LET YOURSELF LAUGH

1. Invite some friends to join you — the more, the merrier. Arrange yourselves on the floor so that you're lying at right angles to each other, one woman's head resting on the next woman's belly. (The first woman in the chain will have her head on the floor; have a pillow handy for her.)

2. The first woman says "Ha!" The next woman adds another "Ha!" and so do the next and the next, passing the lengthening roll of ha-ha's down the chain.

3. If, for some reason, you aren't all breaking up into belly laughs, start trading your bawdiest jokes.

4. Be sure to play a number of rounds, changing places so that the first woman has a chance to be in the middle of the chain.

GLOWING GLOBE

1. Sit comfortably, resting your palms lightly on your lower abdomen. Allowing your breath to deepen into your belly, enter into the Centering Breath.

2. As you breathe, notice the images and sensations occurring within your belly. See and feel the life force focused within your belly center as a glowing sphere of radiant energy. Notice its color: perhaps it's gold, red-orange, ruby red, vermilion, or crimson. Sense its motion: perhaps it's spinning, vibrating, pulsing, or tingling.

3. As you inhale and your belly expands, see and feel how the incoming breath brightens the color of the glowing sphere, making it more potent and vivid. As you exhale and your belly sinks back toward your spine, see and feel how the outgoing breath quickens the sphere, accelerating its spinning, vibrating, pulsing, or tingling.

4. Closing your eyes, take a few moments to experience the images and sensations occurring in the core of your body.

5. Gradually return your awareness to this time and place.

THE POWER OF HOLDING SPACE

This figure holds a bowl in her lap. The bowl *is* her lap.

The bowl is the capacity to receive, to make space for. The first artifact of human culture was likely a container to hold what women were gathering and carrying. Containers — bowls, bags,

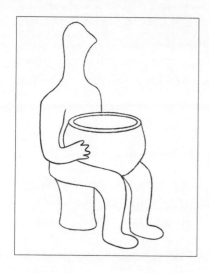

Chevrons mark the back of this clay figurine. Würzburg, Germany, 5500–5200 B.C.E.

basins, baskets, chalices, vases, cauldrons — make it possible to collect water and food, substances vital to life.

The belly, like the bowl, holds space. It's the realm of creative possibility, the fertile void that gives birth to form. It's the cauldron that gathers and concentrates the life force, from which new life emerges. The word *belly* derives from the Old English *belg*. The early meanings of *belg* included "bag," "pod," "the body as the container of the soul," and "uterus."

Your power to promote creation is the power to hold space, to make room, to create an environment that invites wisdom to emerge. When you hold space, you're not trying to make something happen. You're not forcing a particular outcome. You're providing the container for elements to mix and mingle, for possibilities to meet one another and make themselves known. Rather than busily going down your "to do" list, you're attending to what *is*. You're the host receiving the guest, the lover receiving the beloved, the soil receiving the seed.

Your belly-centered power to promote creation is your power to hold space. How do you make room for possibilities to emerge in your life?

THE GOLD-RIMMED BOWL

The bowl is a potent image of the belly as creative space. This image emerged in conversation with a woman who'd had three cesarean sections. "People say I have a 'zipper belly,'" she told me.

As she placed her hand over her belly and let her breath deepen, she reported, "The image that comes up is a coat, a large trench coat with wide lapels and a long double row of buttons. The coat is over a giant zipper. I'm afraid that all my innards will fall out, that they'll leak all over the place."

I suggested she ask her belly what it needed to keep all her innards contained, to keep them from leaking out. As pictures in her mind shifted the way they do in dreams, she answered, "The image that I get is my pelvis as a bowl, a white porcelain bowl with a gold rim. Even though it's porcelain, it's not breakable; it's sacred. There's lots of light coming in on one side, illuminating the front of the bowl. The half that's in back is in shadow."

Bowls, like our bellies, have the capacity to contain apparent opposites — joy and grief, birth and death, light and shadow — and embrace them as complements. Within that embrace, we experience wholeness.

BELLY BOWL

Repeat five times in each direction, with the Centering Breath.

1. Taking a wide stance, place your feet two to three feet apart. Point your toes outward at a comfortable angle. Keeping your knees unlocked, bend them directly over your toes. Keep your weight evenly distributed on your feet. Place your hands lightly on your hips.

2. Gently tilt your pelvis forward.

3. Then tilt your pelvis backward; avoid overarching your lower back. Let your head and neck move naturally toward and away from your chest as your pelvis tilts forward and back.

4. Keeping your knees over your toes, press one hip forward.

5. Then, press your other hip forward. Notice how your knee moves farther out over your toes as the corresponding hip presses forward. Let your head and neck move naturally from side to side as your hips alternate in pressing forward.

6. Still keeping your knees over your toes, roll your pelvis in a slow, full circle.

7. Coming to stillness, rest your palms over your belly center. Notice and feel whatever images and sensations are occurring in your body.

Breath and image: Applying the Centering Breath, inhale during one phase of the motion or one arc of the rotation, exhale during the other. As you tilt and rotate your pelvis, imagine

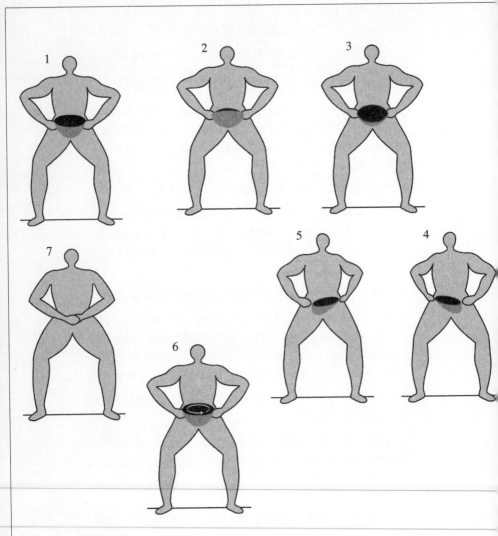

Belly Bowl

your belly as a bowl that contains the elixir of life. Sense how you're stirring the liquid light of your sexual, sensual energy within the bowl that is your belly.

Questions for reflection: What pleasures are you willing to receive? What possibilities do you have a passion to create?

Chapter Eight

Confidence:
Activate Your Self-Assurance

"That took guts." Remember a time when those words could describe something you did, a time when you demonstrated courage and a can-do attitude. Whatever the situation, chances are that you were standing proudly, walking briskly, speaking with animation, looking directly at the person you were addressing.

You were dynamic. You showed that you were ready, willing, and able to act energetically in a purposeful way.

The Shield Yourself in Style and Sing a Proud Song exercises affirm your courage and confidence, making these qualities all the more evident with visual symbols and sound. Concentrating *Hara* Energy adds more "oomph" to your belly breathing. The Power Centering exercise mobilizes the source of your strength, which is deeper than muscle, deeper than willpower. And the Push-Overs exercise enables you to experience how recharging your *hara* steadies your standing in the world.

A woman who works as a blacksmith — and often lifts heavy supplies — says, "I'm using Power Centering every day in the shop. Anytime I'm going to lift something, I do the Power Centering move and grab the energy and pull it in, and it's no problem to move stuff. I've taught it to everyone who's going to lift something. 'Just wait a minute,' I say, 'we've got to do something first here.' And here we are, grabbing up all this energy with Power Centering, and it's so much easier when we have to lift something."

> After a month of struggling with intense lower back pain, job-related depression, confusion, low energy, and no motivation, I woke up one morning and did my belly exercises. I felt energy, strength, and power throughout the day and into the evening. I had been dragging myself to work and coming home feeling exhausted. Now I feel energized and alert. I look forward to new horizons with a high-charge drive coming from within. This is powerful stuff!
>
> — Patty

CONFIDENCE-BOOSTING EXERCISES

If you were a warrior in centuries past, your shield would serve you in several ways. As a barrier to swords and spears, it would protect your belly's vital organs from injury. Decorated with symbols invoking supernatural powers, it would warn away attackers. Marked with signs of your ancestry, it would declare your membership in a family or tribe.

Even if you don't have to engage in hand-to-hand combat in your daily life, you still might want to make an abdominal shield for yourself. As you create it, whether or not you'll ever wear it in public, you claim your right to set boundaries, be safe, and be yourself.

If we don't shield our bellies with our self-validation, we may find that rigid abdominal muscles or extra layers of fat are doing the job for us. As we take responsibility for protecting ourselves and envelop ourselves in self-affirmation, we no longer need that kind of armoring.

> This practice has taken a place that has felt tight and suppressed and shameful, and spoken to that place as a mother nurtures and cradles a child, growing that child into a feeling, functional, and powerful woman.
>
> — Joan

SHIELD YOURSELF IN STYLE

1. Gather your supplies. Choose what you will use as the base for your shield. Possibilities include posterboard, paper plates, a pizza pan, the lid of a large container. Equip yourself with glue, scissors, colored paper, markers, crayons, glitter, stickers, pictures from magazines, ribbons, string, feathers, fabric, leather, beads, gemstones, and the like.

2. Notice any words and images that come to mind as you consider what you want the shield to do for you. How will it serve you? When and how will it come in handy?

3. Enter into the Centering Breath. Notice the words and images that come to mind as you consider the following:

◉   What protects me from injury?

◉   What wards off attack?

◉   What keeps me safe?

◉   What shows my courage?

◉   What tells the world who I am?

Let the emerging words and images guide your design.

4.   When you've completed the shield's design, create a way to hold or wear it in front of your belly. Some possibilities:

◉   Add a handhold to the back of the shield.

◉   Make holes in the shield's side edges and lace a ribbon through the holes in each side. Tie the ribbon behind your back and wear the shield like a low belt over your belly.

◉   Make holes in the shield's top edge. Loop a ribbon through the holes and tie the string around your waist, letting the shield hang down over your belly.

5.   Wearing or holding your shield in place, go to a mirror and appreciate what you see: a woman secure in her self-validation.

There's nothing like belting out a song at maximum volume to amp up your self-assurance. Sing a song in praise of your belly with fingers snapping, hips swinging, and heels tapping. All the elements build on each other — breath, voice, rhythm, rhyme, melody, gesture. Before you know it, you're singing out an anthem for the nation of belly-proud women who've got body confidence to spare!

SING A PROUD SONG

Fit these words to the tune of "Amazing Grace." What other verses can you add?

> *Amazing grace, my belly is round.*
> *It contains my soul's delight.*
> *I once was lost, and now I am found*
> *In the truth that my belly's all right.*

Here's a good-natured parody of Willie Dixon's song "Built for Comfort." Sing these words to your own twelve-bar blues. Or listen to Taj Mahal's rendition of the song on the collection *In Progress & In Motion* (Sony 1998) for some musical ideas. Substitute your own words for "beautiful" and "creation" in the third and fifth lines to make additional verses.

> *Don't try to make my belly thin!*
> *Don't try to make my belly flat!*
> *You better believe my belly's beautiful,*
> *Don't you ever call me fat.*
> *Because I'm built for creation,*
> *I ain't built for speed.*
> *Well, my belly's got everything*
> *This woman needs.*

PUSH-OVERS

Now's your chance to work with a partner in the process of magnifying your confidence. The following exercise draws on the belly-energizing skills you're building — especially Power Centering (see pages 180–83) — and demonstrates some immediate benefits of activating your *hara*. As one woman remarks, "When I'm in my *hara*, I'm grounded in self-love. Self-love is the best self-defense."

Before you begin this exercise, face your partner, standing about an arm's length apart from her. Decide who will go first as "Pusher"; the other person will be "Steadfast." In this experiment, Pusher will reach one arm directly across to Steadfast, and with a firm (but not violent or hurtful) push against her partner's shoulder, attempt to move her backward and off balance.

1. The first step is to calibrate the force of Pusher's push so that it's challenging and still manageable for Steadfast. Pusher offers a few different pushes, pressing against Steadfast's shoulder with varying degrees of firmness. Steadfast tells Pusher what kind of contact is strong enough to be challenging without being jarring or intrusive. Pusher uses that kind of contact in the encounters that follow. Steadfast's job is to stand in place in each of the following three variations.

2. First Variation: Steadfast lets her attention wander before and while Pusher is pressing into her shoulder. She looks up to the ceiling, thinks about what she'll have for

dinner, thinks about her last vacation — she's anything but present in the here and now. She embodies the statement "I'm somewhere else."

3. Second Variation: Steadfast stiffens herself in preparation for Pusher's impending contact. Even before Pusher reaches out, she makes her whole body rigid and tense, making fists with her hands, locking her elbows and knees, gripping the floor with her toes, setting her jaw hard and tight. She embodies the statement "I won't let you get to me."

4. Third Variation: In preparation for the third attempt, Steadfast practices a few rounds of Power Centering. Then, as she faces Pusher, she takes a wide stance, bending her knees over her toes and directing the base of her spine down toward the center of the earth. She breathes slowly and deeply into her belly. With each inhalation she sees and feels the *hara* energy in her belly intensifying and expanding. With each exhalation she sees and feels her *hara* energy streaming down through her legs and into the ground, planting her feet deep into the earth. She looks directly forward as Pusher reaches out to press her shoulder. She embodies the statement "I am here."

5. Repeat each variation several times so that both Pusher and Steadfast can feel what's happening in each attempt and can compare the differences in experience and sensation.

6.   Reverse roles and repeat the experiment several times in each of the three variations.

What do you notice? As Steadfast, in which variation were you least stable, most easily knocked off balance? What were your thoughts and feelings in each one? How did your body move in each one? What was the relationship between your upper body and your lower body in the different variations? Did you notice any relationship between rigidity and instability? Between flexibility and poise? How does this experience relate to events in your life?

As Pusher, in which variation could you most easily shove Steadfast off balance? What were your thoughts and feelings in each attempt? In which variation did you find your interaction with Steadfast most satisfying? How does this experience relate to events in your life?

CONCENTRATING *HARA* ENERGY

1.   Sit comfortably, resting your palms lightly on your lower abdomen. Allow your breath to deepen into your belly, entering into the Centering Breath.

2.   As in the Glowing Globe exercise outlined in chapter 7, see and feel the life force focused within your belly center as a radiant sphere of energy. Notice its color, its motion.

3.   As you inhale, see and feel your breath sinking down into your belly. With your exhalation, gently yet firmly press your belly in toward your spine. See and feel how that pressure

condenses and consolidates your *hara* energy, intensifying the color and the motion of the glowing sphere within your belly center.

4. Closing your eyes, take a few moments to experience the images and sensations occurring in the core of your body.

5. Gradually return your awareness to this time and place.

THE POWER OF NOURISHING

Shapes similar to the seed forms depicted on the next page appear on cave walls, stone monuments, and ceramic vases as well as on big-bellied female figurines.

Shown on its side, the seed form curls around its center point, the point through which nutrients from the surrounding fruit enter its interior. Turned face-up, its shape would be the dot-in-circle. The seed is a map for regeneration, inviting the life force abundant in the universe to enter, infuse, and animate a new form in the process of rebirth.

Your power to promote creation is your capacity to receive nourishment, your willingness to replenish yourself. Nutritious food, clear air, pure water, refreshing movement, invigorating breath, adventuresome play, and deep rest all recharge the vital energy concentrated in your body's core.

Your power to promote creation is also your power to nourish others. When you are full to overflowing with vitality that streams from your body's core, you can effortlessly pay attention to, encourage, and inspire others.

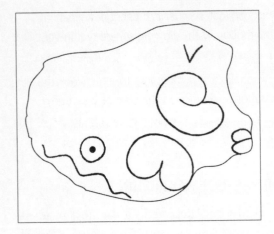

Engravings on this stone, perhaps originally part of a complex tomb site, show seed forms together with a chevron and dot-in-circle. Meath, Ireland, c. 4800 B.C.E.

How and when are you comfortable with giving, with receiving? Are you willing to be all the more generous and receptive in nourishing yourself?

As you move through Power Centering, feel yourself encompassed by an ocean of energy. Let your belly admit an abundant stream of life force directly into your core.

POWER CENTERING

Repeat three times for each position of the arms, with the Energizing Breath.

1. Taking a wide stance, place your feet two to three feet apart. Point your toes outward at a comfortable angle. Keeping your knees unlocked and slightly bent, position them directly over your toes. Place your fists on your hips, palms facing upward.

2. As you inhale, reach both arms straight forward, opening your palms to face downward and extending your fingers forward. Your knees will straighten and your legs will lengthen a bit as you do so.

3. As you exhale through your open mouth, bend your knees and return your hands to your hips. Close your hands into loose fists and rest them lightly on your hips with palms facing upward.

4. Inhaling, raise your arms and open your palms to reach upward at a forty-five-degree angle. Your knees will straighten and your legs will lengthen a bit as you do so.

5. Exhaling through your open mouth and bending your knees, return your hands to your hips in loose fists. Rest them on your hips with palms facing upward.

6. Inhaling, raise your arms and open your palms to reach straight upward. Your knees will straighten and your legs will lengthen a bit as you do so.

7. Exhaling through your open mouth and bending your knees, return your hands to your hips in loose fists. Rest them on your hips with palms facing upward.

8. Inhaling, raise your arms and open your palms to reach upward at a forty-five-degree angle. Your knees will straighten and your legs will lengthen a bit as you do so.

9. Exhaling through your open mouth and bending your knees, return your hands to your hips in loose fists. Rest them on your hips with palms facing upward.

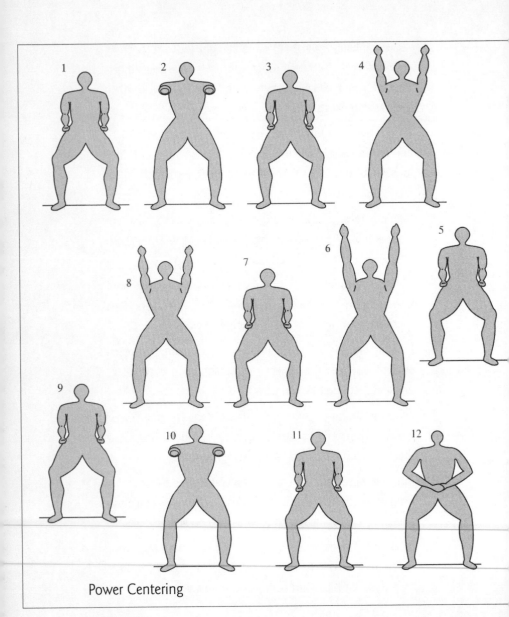

Power Centering

10. Inhaling, open your palms and reach both arms straight forward. Your knees will straighten and your legs will lengthen a bit as you do so.

11. Exhaling through your open mouth and bending your knees, return your hands to your hips in loose fists. Rest them on your hips with palms facing upward.

12. End by returning your palms to rest over your belly center. Notice and feel any images and sensations that are occurring in your body.

Breath and image: Applying the Energizing Breath, inhale as your arms reach out; you're reaching out into an ocean of life energy and claiming a portion of it for yourself. Exhale through your open mouth as your hands return to your hips; you're storing this energy within your body's center.

Question for reflection: How do you choose to nourish yourself?

Chapter Nine

Compassion:
Fill Your Heart to Overflowing

What is love? Perhaps it's giving your attention and compassion freely to another, not expecting anything in return. If that's true, then loving another goes hand in hand with loving yourself. Neglect yourself, and it's easy to start expecting others to fill in for you. Perhaps love is energy moving through the heart, moving with such extravagance that it fills your own heart and spills over, flowing effortlessly out to others.

With the Wish Yourself Well and Honor Your Biography exercises, you can begin developing compassion, even gratitude, for your body's center, no matter how you might have neglected or devalued it in the past. Circle of *Hara* and Heart makes an energetic connection between your heart of creation and your heart of compassion.

Energizing your belly with Lily endows you with endurance, enabling you to love and to keep on loving. One woman relates, "Lily affirms my connection to the natural power of women, to respect for that power. I feel my pelvis open wide, my legs strengthen, my back align. My arms stretch out to embrace life's challenges. Returning to squatting, I reconnect, begin again. Strengthened, aware of myself and my body, I know that the source of my power is within me."

The other day a friend said to me, "You talk from your guts." I like that she noticed. It's true. What I've come to realize, with the help of this practice, is: I am what I've been waiting for.

— Mimi

HEART-OPENING EXERCISES

Our bodies are sentient beings. They feel, sense, learn — and listen. When we bless ourselves, when we bless any part of our bodies, we encourage life energy to flow more freely. Given kind regard, given benevolent attention, we and our bodies flourish.

WISH YOURSELF WELL

When you wish your belly well, you bring your body's center all the more to life.

1. Sit or stand comfortably, or lie on your back with a pillow under your knees to ease your lower back.

2. Enter into the Centering Breath. Place your hands upon your belly, resting them gently over your belly's center.

3. As you breathe, notice any sensations taking place within your belly. You might feel, for example, sensations of temperature, density, texture, vibration, or motion.

4. As you breathe, notice any images that appear. Perhaps there are colors, shapes, or lines coming into your awareness.

5. Listen, too, for sounds. There may be melodies, words or phrases, a story, descriptions, or even messages.

6. Just notice what's true for you, however subtle, however obvious. There's no right or wrong way to do this. In your own unique way, you are contacting something of the mystery, something of the potency, that's alive within the interior of your belly.

7. Sense that your palms can actually transmit a message. You might imagine the surface of your hands emitting a light or warmth or vibration that penetrates deeply into your belly, carrying a message along with it.

8. With your own words and images, send a message all the way through to your belly's center, wishing it well. Continue transmitting your message for ten or more cycles of breathing.

I was tired, distressed, and down on myself, with that nasty commentator replaying negative messages over and over in my brain. After doing the belly exercises, I felt empowered, centered, energized — and light. Breath of fire, of life, of joy.

— Tricia

9. As your palms send your message, notice how your belly responds. Notice any shifts in inner image or sensation or sound.

10. When you feel satisfied that your message has been sent and received, simply return your awareness to your breath. Then slowly expand your awareness into your entire body, and into the present moment.

How did your belly respond to your wish for its well-being?
What impressions, insights, or understandings emerged for you
in this experience?

One woman wrote a poem to describe the images and sensations of her body's center and how they shifted in response to her expression of caring:

SANCTUARY

Glowing globe,
red warm belly center of me —
I soothe and comfort you,
guard and shelter.
What do I say to you?
"You are safe here
 inside."

In response
it shimmers,
it lotuses,
it galaxies into life.

— Carol Barre

One powerful way to reshape the way you feel and think about your belly is to consider its history. Appreciating your belly's biography equips you to reinvent your relationship with your body's center and make it mutually rewarding.

Your belly contains worlds of experience — laughter and grief, pleasure and pain, confusion and certainty, challenge and triumph. Your belly's biography both shapes and reveals its biology.

Be gentle and respectful as you discover your belly's personal history. In many ways our culture "can't stomach" a woman's belly. Whether we're awake to it or not, that rejection is painful. We often cope with the culture's rejection by cooperating with it — by scorning our bellies, numbing our core feelings, and denying our instinctive knowing. We try to protect ourselves as well as we can.

When we cooperate with the culture's rejection, however, we repress our sense of self. We muffle our inner authority, guidance, and purpose. We mute our creativity. We restrict our sexual expression.

As you listen to your belly's stories and honor its biography, you create a more compassionate relationship with your belly. At the same time, you can reclaim an expanded sense of who you are.

HONOR YOUR BIOGRAPHY

This exercise draws on the inspiration of Ira Progoff's *At a Journal Workshop*.¹ Follow these steps to elicit your belly's biography:

1. What events have shaped how you think and feel about your belly? Consider the stages of your life. What did you experience as a child, a preteen, and a teenager that formed your relationship with your belly? What have you experienced as an adult? Jot down a quick word or phrase to note each event, listing these experiences as you remember

them, whatever their actual sequence in time. To stir your memory, consider the following:

Beginnings:

What was your first awareness of your belly?

What was your first feeling about your belly?

What's the first thing someone said to you about your belly?

When (if ever) did you stop breathing deeply? What was happening in your life at that time?

When (if ever) did you start feeling ashamed of your belly? What was happening in your life at that time?

Words and images:

What have your family and friends said about your belly — and about theirs?

What words have you used to speak about your belly?

What magazines, movies, TV shows, and celebrities have influenced how you think and feel about your belly?

Experiences:

What has your belly been through in relation to any of the following?

- food, eating, mealtimes, diets, digestion, elimination

- illness, injuries, accidents, surgery, healing

- clothes, weight loss, weight gain, body size, body shape

- menstruation, PMS, birth control

- dating, sex, pregnancy, childbirth, menopause
- exercise, sports, dance, holidays
- creative expression
- intuition, inner guidance, "gut feelings"

2. When your list is complete, mark each event with the year in which it occurred. Now number the events according to their sequence in time. Rewrite the list, arranging the events in chronological order — from the most distant in time to the most recent.

3. Look for the thread that links these moments together. Is there a theme? Is there a way in which your experience has been developing? Write a few sentences summarizing and reflecting upon what you see.

4. Look for two or three experiences that were turning points in your relationship with your belly. Develop your notes on these events further, telling the whole story. What more can you say about these events now, given your current perspective?

One woman recalls:

1st or 2nd grade, 6 yrs old: Little boy I liked elbowed me in the belly. It hurt so bad. . . . I couldn't breathe, and just as much, my feelings were hurt. We never really laughed together after that.

9–10 yrs old: My father talked about how hard my stomach was: "No flab on her." He was very complimentary about it and poked his own belly saying how it wasn't so firm anymore.

20 yrs old: Very thin . . . until I put on a little weight in my early twenties. Nobody had ever seen me with any padding and they commented . . . and I felt very dowdy and unattractive and pudgy. . . .

Another woman notes:

16 yrs old: Ate so much at Thanksgiving had to lie down.
24 yrs old: First good sexual experience — very freeing.
29 yrs old: C-section; I felt torn apart.

And another recalls:

I've always been embarrassed about my "wub" — that's what we called our bellies in high school if they stuck out at all.

CIRCLE OF *HARA* AND HEART

1. Sit or lie comfortably. Allow your breath to deepen into your belly, and enter into the Centering Breath. Rest your right hand over your lower abdomen and place your left hand on the center of your chest.

2. Focus on breathing into your *hara*, then circle the breath up through your chest and breathe out through your heart. See and feel a circuit of breath and energy connecting your *hara* and your heart.

3. Closing your eyes, take a few moments to experience the images and sensations occurring in your body.

4. Gradually return your awareness to this time and place.

THE POWER OF RENEWING

The lily is an ancient symbol of rebirth, one we see on grave markers as well as at Easter, invoking life's return from death.

Your power to promote creation is the power of renewing and regenerating. Cycles proceed through beginning, middle, and end. Then what? The moon moves through phases of waxing, full, and waning. Then what? The seasons move from spring to summer to fall. Then what?

The stillness of winter allows seeds to germinate and leaves to unfurl from their buds come spring. The new moon's darkness prepares the way for the increase of light. The nothingness beyond the end is the fertile void — the silence, the blankness — that yields another beginning.

When you allow yourself to be still, to be silent, to rest, you're invoking your capacity for renewal. Putting aside your list of things to do, you're allowing yourself simply to be. Releasing judgment and expectations, you return to and rest in the center of who you are. The fountain of life energy springing from your body's center replenishes and rejuvenates you.

When and how do you allow yourself to rest? In what ways do you cultivate stillness and silence?

As you move through Lily, rising from squatting into standing with arms outstretched, feel yourself to be a lily flowering into full

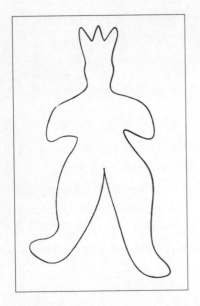

A lily springs from the head of this terra-cotta figurine. Thessaly, Greece, c. 6000 B.C.E.

bloom. As you return to squatting, folding your arms inward, feel yourself returning to the earth and into seed form, preparing for yet another round of renewal.

LILY

Repeat seven times, with the Energizing Breath.

1. Taking a wide stance, place your feet two to three feet apart. Point your toes outward at a comfortable angle. Keeping your knees unlocked and slightly bent, position them directly over your toes. Close your hands into loose fists. Bend your elbows and bring your forearms together in front of your chest.

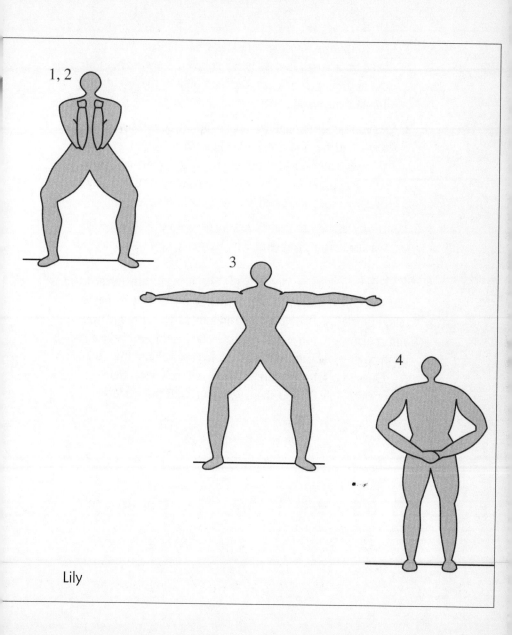

1, 2

3

4

Lily

2. As you inhale, keeping your knees directly over your toes, bend your knees further and sink down a few inches into the beginning of a squat. Descend only to the level that's comfortable for you.

3. As you exhale through your open mouth, squeeze your buttocks together and rise to standing. At the same time, extend your arms straight out to your sides at shoulder level, with your palms facing forward. Keep your knees bent slightly over your toes and avoid arching your lower back.

4. End by resting your palms over your belly center. Notice and feel whatever images and sensations are occurring in your body.

Breath and image: Applying the Energizing Breath, inhale as you sink down: you're reaching down into the earth to gather vitality. Exhale through your open mouth as you rise and your arms open wide: you're drawing this vitality into your belly and up through your heart, sending the overflow out into the world.

Questions for reflection: How do you replenish the love in your heart? How do you share your love with the world?

Chapter Ten

Creativity:
Unleash Your Self-Expression

"When I was pregnant with my children — that's when I felt good about my belly," one woman recalls. A woman's capacity to send new life into the world is magnificent beyond what words can say. A woman's procreative power is not limited to childbirth, however. It is also pro-creative — the power to promote creation in whatever dimension you choose. Your belly is a cauldron of creative energy. You put that energy to use when you generate new kinds of relationships, new enterprises. You use it as you put your vision into action, your ideas into expression. You use it as you enfold what's beautiful and true into forms we can see, hear, taste, smell, and touch.

If you're alive, if you're breathing, you're creative. Creativity is one expression of your life energy as a whole. Your creativity flows freely as you give yourself permission and safety to express yourself.

The Start a Correspondence and Dialogue with Your Inner Wisdom exercises enable you to access the originality of your authentic self. Directing the Breath enables you to guide the flow of Source Energy to any place in your body, dissolving the sense of being sluggish or stuck into the ease of freely streaming creative change.

When you energize your belly with Wings, it takes the wraps off your passion and brings forth your capacity to create. One woman says, "I feel like a bird when I do Wings, as if I'm standing before the ocean on the beach at sunset, feeling the air rush through me, as if I am becoming the tides. I can smell it, hear it, taste it! I had trouble with this one at first; I would step too far back, like a gymnast. Throughout, I've realized that I hold so much tension in my neck and shoulders, and here it's no exception. Letting go of my head, being in my whole body, I move much more smoothly, more gracefully. It does take some thinking and concentration to correctly coordinate my body with the movements, and I'm finding that with repetition and practice I'm able to experience the movements more and more."

This whole program has inspired so much creative work. It's a well for going down into my center and getting whatever images are there. It has helped me to go to where I just see those images. One image that came to me was two worlds coming together, like body and spirit joining in communion. That image is an actual sculpture now. Maybe the significance for me is that finally I'm able to bring spirit into the physical, that it's easier, there's a flow, a constant flow of energy.

— Tekla

CREATIVITY-ENHANCING EXERCISES

Consider your belly to have its own identity, its own personality. You can communicate with this character by writing a letter to your belly.

The idea of your belly having its own voice, feelings, needs, and sense of humor might seem strange. If you've neglected or rejected it, you may be afraid of what your belly might tell you. Actually, you may be surprised by your belly's willingness to forgive and by the strength of its desire to create a loving relationship with you.

> I have a powerful, gutsy belly that will lead me if I will talk and listen to her.
>
> — Susan

START A CORRESPONDENCE

1. Write a letter to your belly.
2. Write down your belly's response.
3. Continue the correspondence as you wish.

Here's an example of one woman's correspondence with her belly. She begins by acknowledging the pain her belly has experienced in the past. She articulates her understanding that the way she thinks affects what her belly feels.

Dear Belly-o-mine:

I know how much discomfort you've been in all these years. Until recently, I haven't believed that I could deliberately choose thoughts that would create something better for us both!

Well, now I know how to do better for you. Just think how much better you and I have felt in the last few months.

What do you think? Do you feel that we are consciously and deliberately choosing what is positive?

Now I know better what a negative or painful feeling coming from you means — it's a signal that I'm focusing on what I don't want.

Sincerely,
Ann

Ann's belly responds with gusto to her invitation to converse. Note the energy and immediacy of her belly's reply. Given the opportunity to speak, Belly voices its central concerns with emotional honesty in direct, no-nonsense terms.

Dear Ann,

Boy! You've been filling me full with food because you haven't known to fill me with your loving attention. This is the nourishment I need. I don't need all the second helpings and recreational tidbits. I need reasonable basics and you. You, meaning your caring attention.

Whether you are prepared to believe it or not, you are important. I cannot go on without you. How long do I have to keep calling out to you while you keep saying, "What? Me? I'm worthless. How could someone be calling out to me?"

I'll die without you and your attention; that makes you important to me. If you say that you don't count, that you can't be important unless you get the attention of parents who are already dead and gone, then there is no hope for me. But I have to believe the truth — that you need me and I love you.

Yours truly,

Belly

Ann's reply demonstrates that she has received Belly's message. In response to Belly's expressed need for her attention, she's willing to value herself in totally new ways. Understanding the importance of her attention to Belly's well-being, she's willing to move to the center of her life, to validate herself. Her response shows transformation in process.

Dear Belly-o-mine,

I truly haven't thought my attention was all that important to you — just as my inattentive parents never would have imagined how vitally important their attention could have been to me as a child.

Not having felt valued, I've found it hard to believe that anything I might do or offer could matter much. You have been crying out in neglect, and I haven't believed that my attention could make any difference. Yet I'm understanding now that I can make all the difference.

How do I know? My Belly told me so.

Love,

Ann

As you and your belly write letters to each other, as in the previous exercise, you're opening an important channel of communication. Engaging in a back-and-forth dialogue makes your communication all the more immediate and intimate.

Again, the idea of speaking to your belly and listening to its reply may seem strange. Understandably, if you've ignored, criticized, or even abused your belly, you might be afraid to hear what it has to say to you. Be open to the possibility that your belly actually craves to have a loving relationship with you.

Activating your belly with movement and breath encourages your belly to communicate with you. If you practice the sequence of belly-energizing exercises, for example, and then do the following Dialogue with Your Inner Wisdom, you're likely to enjoy a lively exchange.

DIALOGUE WITH YOUR INNER WISDOM

Give yourself ample time for this dialogue. Set aside fifteen to twenty minutes during which you'll be free from interruption. Equip yourself with a notebook or stack of paper and a pen or pencil.

Write out the dialogue with your belly as it is taking place. Make a clear distinction between your voice and your belly's voice by asking each party to speak in the first person, addressing the other as "you." For example, you might say to your belly, "I wish you would..." and your belly might say to you, "I like that you...." Expressing each voice distinctly lays the foundation for building a strong and reciprocal relationship.

1. Enter into the Centering Breath and notice any images and sensations that come into your awareness as you focus your attention within your body's center.

2. Begin by inviting conversation. Your belly might not be ready to chat right away. Develop a mutual willingness to talk with a statement like this:

    "Hello! I'd really like to talk with you. Are you willing to speak with me?"

    Don't be surprised if your belly is initially grumpy or skeptical. Let it speak those feelings, or let it be silent for a while as you gently repeat your invitation.

    If your belly doesn't answer you at first in words, it may respond with a shift in inner sensation and imagery. Demonstrate your patience, your willingness to be with your belly and treat it with respect.

3. Make introductions. Ask your belly its name:

    "What do you want me to call you?"

    Use that name to address your belly throughout your conversation. One woman's belly was Giver of Life; another's was Belle.

4. Stay present. As you write, be totally honest about what's happening in the moment. There's no need to be polite, smart, or quick with this process. Express exactly what's true for you.

    For example, if you're afraid that you don't know how to talk to your belly, write something like this:

    "Belly, I'm afraid I don't know how to talk to you."

    If you're worried that your belly is so angry about all the ways you've mistreated it in the past that it won't want to talk with you, write this:

"Belly, I'm worried that you're so angry with me for all the ways I've mistreated you in the past that you won't want to talk with me."

5. Attend to feelings. Listen to your belly's feelings, and then express your own. Invite your belly to tell you how it feels with words such as:

    "Please tell me how you're feeling. I'm ready and willing to listen to whatever you have to say to me. I want to hear it all."

    Invite your belly to express itself fully. When it comes to a stop, you might say this:

    "What else? What else do you want to tell me about how you're feeling?"

    When it's your turn to express your feelings, tell the complete truth.

6. Attend to needs. Listen and respond to your belly's needs, and then express your own. When you ask your belly what it needs from you, get the specifics.

    If your belly says, "I need you to be nice to me," keep asking for the details until it tells you, for example, "I need you to sit down when you eat. I need you to turn the television off. I need you to chew your food really well."

    If you can't or don't want to meet the need that your belly has stated, say so:

    "I don't know how to do that." Or, "That's boring. I'm not willing to do that."

    You may also want to ask, "Will you help me find a way to do that?"

    When it's your turn, tell the complete truth. And ask whether and how your belly can address your needs.

7. Express your gratitude to each other. Tell your belly what you truly appreciate about it. Listen to your belly appreciating you. Make your appreciation sincere. Find something, anything, that sparks the feeling of gratitude for each of you.

   You might say, "Belly, with all the discomfort you've caused me, you've made me realize that I need to take better care of myself in many ways. I'm grateful to you for that."

   Your belly might say, "I appreciate that you're paying attention to me."

8. Make promises to each other that you both will keep. A simple, small, very specific promise will do.

   You might say, "Belly, I promise that at least one day a week I will eat breakfast sitting down."

   Your belly might say, "I promise I'll talk to you in this kind of conversation rather than getting indigestion to get your attention."

9. Agree — and promise — to meet and talk again. Arrange a specific time and place to continue your conversation. Your belly needs to know that you are trustworthy. If you make a promise to your belly, plan to keep it.

If you're addressing a complex situation, you may need to engage your belly in several conversations and keep a series of promises before your belly is willing to communicate freely and fully. The way I see it, the body is incredibly forgiving. Still, if there's a history of neglect or miscommunication, your first priority is rebuilding trust.

DIRECTING THE BREATH

1. Sit or lie comfortably. Allow your breath to deepen into your belly, and enter into the Centering Breath.

2. As you breathe, notice the images and sensations occurring within your belly. See and feel the life energy focused within your belly center growing brighter and stronger with each breath.

3. Breathing in through your *hara*, send the breath from your *hara* to any area in your body that needs warmth, energy, attention, or healing, and breathe out through that place. (As attention and energy return to a site that's been numb or injured, the sensations that accompany the increased awareness may be a bit uncomfortable. Go slowly, with the intention to witness rather than resist sensation. Your breath and your compassionate awareness will encourage the process of healing.)

4. Closing your eyes, take a few moments to experience the images and sensations occurring in the area through which the breath is flowing.

5. Gradually return your awareness to this time and place.

THE POWER OF EXPRESSING

Bird-shaped icons and other figures with birdlike beaks and masks are found as cave wall engravings, small clay and stone statues, and ceramic vases and urns. The chevron recalls the sight of birds in flight.

The winged creature conveys both life and death. To this day, we picture the stork as delivering babies out of the blue. Owls, vultures, crows, and other birds remind us of the passage into the realm beyond life.

Birds move fluidly through regions of water and air. They move between the visible and the invisible, the known and the unknown. They carry the news from heaven to earth and back again.

Your power to promote creation is the power of expressing, giving voice to your gut-level knowing. Expressing yourself takes your wisdom out into the world, unearths it, brings it to light.

The creative energy concentrated in your core wants and needs to move. As you express yourself, your originality, your authenticity, you're participating in the cycle of giving and receiving. The world nourishes you with food, water, air, and friendship.

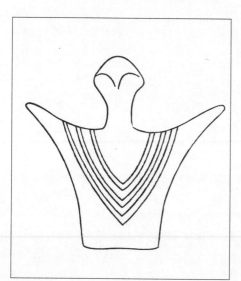

Triple chevrons decorate this winged figure. Moravia, c. 5000 B.C.E.

Sharing your creativity with the world, you're returning these gifts in kind.

What's more, the world needs to see, hear, and feel what you're discovering to be true. The creative power within your core is your instinct for self-preservation, both as an individual and as a member of the human tribe. The expression of your creativity contributes to our well-being, our survival, as a whole.

When you give voice to your truth, you're putting your continuing process of discovery into images, gestures, and words. You're inviting your creative spirit into form, making it available for others to appreciate.

When and how do you enjoy expressing yourself? What would inspire, encourage, and support your process of self-expression?

As you move through Wings, feel yourself embodying the birdlike capacity both to soar upward and to swoop downward, to bring heaven down to earth, and to bring the regenerating gifts of life into the here and now, into the receptivity of your body's center.

WINGS

Repeat three times, with the Energizing Breath.

1.　Stand with your feet parallel to each other, hip-width apart. Bend your knees slightly, keeping them directly over your toes. Lengthen your arms alongside your body.

2.　If you prefer, keep your feet in place. Otherwise, bend your knees further and shift your weight into your left foot. Inhaling,

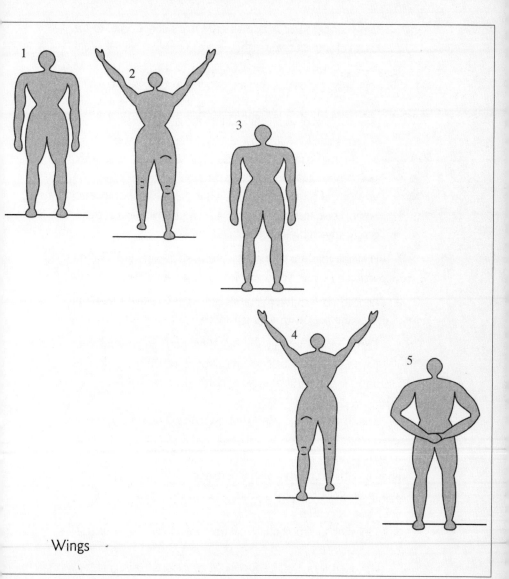

Wings

step your right foot back a distance that's about equal to the length of your foot; your right toes point nearly straight forward as they angle out only a few degrees to the right. Distribute your weight evenly upon your two feet as both of your knees remain bent. Keeping both hips and knees pointing forward, press the heel of your right foot into the ground. Press the base of your spine forward to avoid overarching your lower back.

At the same time as you step your right foot back, sweep both arms forward, up, and out into the shape of a V. With arms stretched out, your palms are facing each other. Look forward and up, at a forty-five-degree angle, gently stretching your chest and throat.

3. Exhaling through your open mouth, step your right foot forward and sweep your arms forward and down to your sides.

4. Repeat, now shifting your weight onto your right foot and stepping back with your left foot.

5. Come to stillness in the standing position, resting your palms over your belly center. Notice and feel any images and sensations occurring in your body.

Breath and image: Applying the Energizing Breath, inhale as you reach your arms up and out; you're opening your wings to soar, sending forth your self-expression. Exhale through your open mouth as you step your feet together and return your arms alongside your body; you're resting in the creative power of your body's center.

Question for reflection: What truth are you willing to express?

Chapter Eleven

Intuition:
Amplify Your Inner Guidance

"Trust your gut." A friend might use these words to encourage you to follow your inner guidance. The words point to the link between your belly and your intuition.

How do you know what your gut instincts are telling you? Here are three ways my belly guides me:

- If I center my awareness in my belly and ask myself "What will happen if I. . .?" an image comes to mind that gives me an idea of the consequences.

- If I focus my awareness in my belly as I'm considering my options, my belly tenses up as I think of one choice and relaxes as I think of another.

◈   When I'm writing in my journal about an issue
    that's been troubling me and come to a resolution,
    my belly rumbles, affirming my insight out loud!

Mixed with a multitude of hopes and fears, your gut feelings
may seem muddled. Use the Stay in Touch and Draw Out Your
Deepest Knowing exercises to clarify your inner wisdom, to become all the more aware of your intuitive know-
ing. Breathing into heaven and earth amplifies
your sense of receiving both information and
support.

When I am
centered in my body, I feel a
solid foundation under my life.
I feel as if I have an inner guidance
system constantly at work in all decisions I make, both large and
small. I know what to do.

— *Connie*

Practicing the Tree focuses your attention within your body's center, quieting
the mind's chaotic chatter and turning up the
volume on your inner knowing. One woman
writes, "I am enjoying the Tree. I feel so grounded,
yet suspended, or perhaps elongated. Like a prism,
I'm attracting energy from the sky, as well as pulling energy up
from the earth, all in touch and in tune with the belly center, res-
onating from the belly."

INTUITION-BUILDING EXERCISES

Rubbing your tummy feels good. The gentle massage in the exercise that follows leads you back to feeling calm, relaxed, and reas-
sured. It's a wonderful method of self-care that makes you all the
more receptive to your inner guidance.

You might invite a trusted friend to share this experience with you, trading gentle tummy rubs. Touching a woman's belly — your own or another's — is a profoundly moving experience. You're touching the essence of life. Take time to bring awareness, respect, and appreciation to the experience.

STAY IN TOUCH

Here's how to give your tummy a pleasing massage:

1. Make yourself comfortable by lying down on a well-padded surface. Place your feet flat on the ground, keeping your knees bent. Support your knees by placing pillows underneath them.

2. Enter into the Centering Breath.

3. Place your palm gently upon your navel. Slowly glide your hand in clockwise circles, spiraling outward to cover the whole surface of your belly.

4. As your hand circles, see and feel comforting light and soothing warmth penetrating deeply.

5. Still moving your hand in a clockwise direction, spiral in toward your navel. Slowly bring your hand to stillness over your navel and let it rest there for a few moments. Enjoy the sense of relaxation you've evoked. Remain open to sensations and images that carry your instinctive wisdom into your awareness.

"Trusting your gut" means using your intuition along with your logic and sense of ethics to make a choice or set a course of action. You may be willing to trust your gut, but the guidance your belly is giving you may not come through in neat sentences. Drawing the images that your belly generates can help clarify your gut instincts.

You may have been told at a tender age that you weren't creative, that you couldn't draw. If that's the case, here's good news: what you're about to do is not Fine Arts 101. If anything, what you need is a *Romper Room* mentality — have fun making a mess. I use the word *drawing* as code for holding a colored marker in your hand and moving it around the paper with abandon. You won't be graded or judged. You don't have to make the page look good for anyone, not even yourself. There's no right or wrong way to do this kind of doodling. There's no such thing as a mistake. Feel your way into it, play around with it, surprise yourself.

DRAW OUT YOUR DEEPEST KNOWING

1. Get a stack of plain white paper and a set of markers.

2. Sitting comfortably, enter into the Centering Breath. Notice any images and sensations that come into your awareness as you focus your attention within your body's center.

3. Consider your arm to be an extension of your belly, a pipeline ready to carry information from your body's center through to your hand and out onto paper. Maintaining your awareness in your belly, take the markers that appeal to you. Let your arm and hand move across the paper, spilling out colors,

shapes, and lines. Give yourself all the permission you need to make your marks freely, without judgment or restriction.

4. When you sense that your drawing is complete, pause. See whether there's a word or phrase you want to add as a title or a caption. If so, add it to the page in the color and style that feels right to you.

5. If your drawing seems incomplete in some way (or you just want to do more), take a new sheet of paper and make another drawing. Allow yourself to use as much paper as you want. Give yourself full permission — to "make it ugly" or "do it wrong" or "be sloppy" or "make a mess." As you give yourself total freedom of expression, your true picture will emerge.

6. When you've finished, take a moment to regard your picture and receive its message, in the same way that you might appreciate the guidance you receive in a dream. Write the date on your drawing and keep it together with all your drawings in a special place.

You can do belly drawings before and after practicing the sequence of belly-energizing exercises. Drawing a picture before you begin and again after you finish a session may demonstrate the effect that energizing your belly is having on your body and mind.

If you've made before-and-after drawings, sit quietly with the two pictures in front of you, placing "before" on the left and "after" on the right. Notice how the pictures are similar and how they differ. There's no right or wrong. What do the drawings show about the difference that energizing your belly has made for you?

BREATHING INTO HEAVEN AND EARTH

As you breathe into your belly center and direct the breath to and through each place in your body, remain with each location for ten to twenty cycles of the breath.

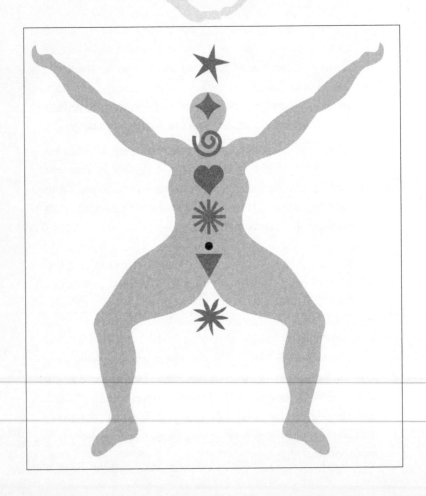

1. Sit comfortably, resting your palms lightly on your lower abdomen. Allowing your breath to deepen into your belly, enter into the Centering Breath.

    As you breathe, notice the images and sensations occurring within your belly. See and feel the life force focused within your belly center. Notice its shape and color; sense its motion; listen for its sounds. See and feel the life energy focused within your belly growing brighter and stronger with each breath.

2. Breathing into your belly center, now breathe out through your perineum and down into the earth.

3. Breathing into your belly center, breathe out through the front and back of your body from the center of your lower abdomen.

4. Breathing into your belly center, breathe out through the front and back of your body from the center of your upper abdomen at a level just beneath your ribs.

5. Breathing into your belly center, breathe out through the front and back of your body from the center of your chest.

6. Breathing into your belly center, breathe out through the front and back of your body from the center of your throat.

7. Breathing into your belly center, breathe out through the front and back of your body from the center of your forehead.

8. Breathing into your belly center, breathe out through your perineum and down into the earth. At the same time, breathe from your belly center out through the crown of your head and up into the heavens.

9. Closing your eyes, take a few moments to experience the images and sensations occurring throughout your body.

10. Gradually return your awareness to this time and place.

THE POWER OF CONNECTING

The tree appears in rock carvings, ceramic designs, and tombs and shrines. It signifies the World Axis, connecting the airy realms with the earth, its roots reaching deeply into the wellspring of all life.

Many cultures have linked the tree to the power to promote creation through words. In Indian tradition, for example, the Mother of the Universe reveals herself as a tree; her leaves bear the signs of the sound vibrations that bring the world into being. Celtic tradition associates each letter of the alphabet with a specific tree. Sequencing leaves on a string or rod spells out a secret message. In some cultures trees were known as the source of oracular wisdom. The word *tree* and the words *truth* and *truce* trace their origin to a common root, the Old English *tréow*.

Your power to promote creation is the power to connect, to reach out to apparently opposing end points and include them in a single embrace. You're dissolving the barrier between elements that have appeared to be mutually exclusive. You're creating a bridge — between light and dark, right and wrong, good and bad, heaven and earth. This is the process of integrating, healing, becoming whole. This is the process of peacemaking.

This is also the process of growth. Imagine a seedling, just beginning to emerge from its shell. From one point, it sinks roots down into the earth. From that same point, it reaches stem and leaves toward the sky.

As you move through the Tree, feel your body both reaching up and sinking down, extending through the worlds of heaven and earth. Feel your body configuring the unity of these realms

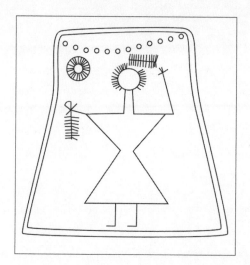

Ceramic design shows
figure with tree branches.
Sardinia, Italy,
c. 4000–3800 B.C.E.

within the totality of life itself. Feel yourself standing in the truth
of who you are.

TREE

Hold each position for ten cycles of the Centering Breath.

1. Stand with your feet parallel, hip-width apart, your knees
    bending slightly over your toes. Lengthen your arms along-
    side your body, with your palms facing your body's midline.
    Focus your gaze — and your mind's eye — on a point
    straight in front of you.

2. If you prefer, keep your heels on the ground. Otherwise, lift
    your heels and roll onto the balls of your feet as you reach
    one arm down and the other forward and up. Feel both

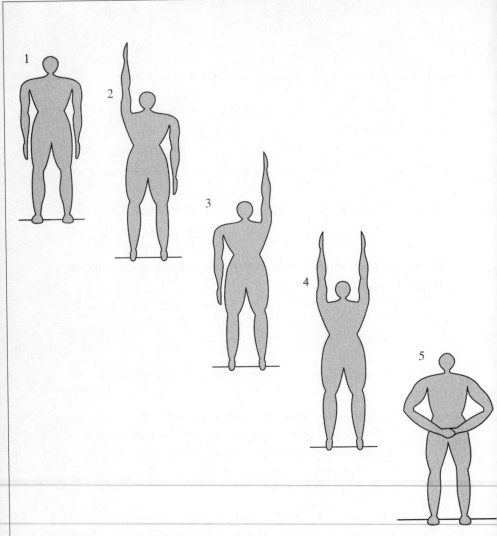

Tree

arms rooted in your belly, stretching out from your body's center. Slowly lower your upraised arm as you slowly return your heels to the ground.

3. Repeat, lifting the opposite arm.

4. Repeat again, raising both arms.

5. Come to stillness, resting your palms over your belly center. Notice and feel any images and sensations occurring in your body.

Breath and image: Applying the Centering Breath, gently stretch out from your center with each inhalation, lengthening upward and downward at the same time. Release the stretch slightly with each exhalation. As you rise onto your toes with your arms stretched overhead, feel the crown of your head reaching into the sky and your feet rooting into the earth. Feel yourself being a tree.

Questions for reflection: How do you expand your reach to connect with and embrace apparent opposites? In what ways are you kin to the trees?

Chapter Twelve

Purpose:
Make Your Dreams Come True

"Follow your heart, live your dream." You might say these words to a friend when you're urging her to be true to herself, to honor her own sense of purpose.

How do you make your dreams into reality? You might begin by wishing upon a star, a lovely image of asking for heavenly help. Next, you clarify your heart's desire. Then you apply your "gut determination" to bring your dream down to earth.

The Picture Your Heart's Desire exercise refines the skill you've already developed in setting your intention and engages your Source Energy in supporting your life purpose. Healing into Wholeness provides a powerful way to resolve conflicts, keeping you on track and moving forward. Focusing and directing your Source Energy with Alignment empowers you to realize your heart's desire and live true to your life's purpose.

One woman writes, "We were doing the Alignment in class one night and an image came to me from my belly. A Native American woman, beautiful, with raven hair; her hand held the hand of a small child. She said to me, 'I am Kiani, which means "two rivers." I will be your connection. I will be your friend. I will be here to help, to answer questions, calm fears, share stories, lives. Come with me. Let us drink from the river, we will braid each other's hair. Our children will play.' Smiling into her eyes, I took her other hand and felt as one with her. This is how profound these belly exercises are, how profoundly this honoring of my belly has helped me. Her culture lives with and respects nature; mine does not. Maybe together we can bridge the chasm, heal."

I have created a lot of energy with this practice. I am so much more focused and am attracting energy to me... envisioning what I want, believing it, and creating. I check in with my belly, asking her, "Does this feel right?"

— Tricia

PURPOSE-DISCERNING EXERCISES

What is your heart's desire? What do you want to be, do, and have that will make your dearest dreams come true? When you connect your gut determination with your heart's desire, you're on your way to making it so.

Remember a time — or make one up — when you wanted something with every particle of your being. You had no doubt about it. You were totally ready to receive it. You were willing to do whatever you needed to do within the bounds of ethical behavior to receive this goodness into your life.

Recall the state of your body. How were you standing, moving, speaking, breathing? What were the sensations in your belly? What emotions were you experiencing? What kinds of excitement were you feeling? That's what I mean by "gut determination."

Gut determination is not about forcing others or straining yourself. It is about cultivating the steadfast certainty that you deserve — and are already in the process of realizing — your heart's desire.

Energizing your belly with movement and breath is one way to develop your gut determination. You can focus this power by picturing your heart's desire.

I had been teaching art in the public schools for twelve years. Getting in touch with my belly gave me the courage I needed to let go. I said, "This is it. I need to be true to what I need to be." After I quit, it seemed as if a burden lifted off my shoulders. Now I'm confident in running my own business. And my art is out there.

— *Tekla*

PICTURE YOUR HEART'S DESIRE

1. Get a stack of plain white paper and some colored markers. Enter into the Centering Breath.

2. As you focus your awareness within your belly, let the knowledge of your heart's desire come to mind. What do you want so much you can practically taste it?

   Keep breathing and focusing within your belly, waiting patiently to receive this knowledge. Your heart's desire may emerge as a visual image, a phrase, or a sensation.

   Check in with your belly as possibilities arise, asking

your inner guidance, "Do I really want this? Am I totally ready and willing to receive this in my life?" Wait until you see, hear, or feel a mighty "Yes!" in your gut.

3. Now, with that *Romper Room* mentality — having fun making a mess — take markers in hand and let lines, shapes, and colors spill out onto paper, allowing an image of your desire to come into view. Use several pieces of paper, as many as you need, to revise the image until you're satisfied it's the picture of your heart's desire.

4. You might prefer to represent your heart's desire with words rather than with a visual image. If so, write a few sentences to describe what's happening and how you feel as your dream comes true. Use your favorite color and style of lettering to put these words onto paper.

Place this image of your heart's desire at eye level on the wall in front of you as you practice the belly-energizing moves, using the image as your visual focus. Experiment with making each of the exercises a gesture that draws this image into your body's center; brighten the image with each breath.

As you practice Tree, for example, notice how focusing your gaze on the image of your heart's desire helps you maintain your balance. As you practice Alignment, notice how this focus strengthens your sense of purpose.

As you sense the image of your heart's desire developing within your belly, envelop the image in your feeling of gut determination. Cultivate a sense of gratitude as well, knowing that the goodness you desire is already on its way into your life. Your clarity of purpose, your gut determination, and your gratitude bring the blessing into being.

Holy, *wholeness*, *hale*, and *healing* are words that stem from the same root. These words suggest that healing occurs through the encounter of opposites: day and night, light and dark, this and that. When polar opposites meet and intermingle, their union generates a more encompassing awareness, an expanded sense of self, an evolution of consciousness, a rebirth.

What are these polar elements? They're often represented as human and divine, masculine and feminine, heaven and earth, good and bad, right and wrong.

As we identify the conflicting needs and desires that are active in our own lives, we name the origin of our own distress and disease. As we allow these apparent opposites to meet and integrate through breath, image, and gesture, we facilitate our own healing. We move into another dimension of wholeness.

HEALING INTO WHOLENESS

1. Take a few moments — through journal writing, meditation, or reflection — to identify some of the conflicting needs and desires operating in your life at this time. Part of you may want to have or do "this," and at the same time another part of you may want to have or do "that." Distinguish the elements of these polarities as clearly as you can.

2. Sitting comfortably, with your back straight and your feet flat on the floor, place your hands on your knees, palms facing upward. Deepen your breath, allowing your belly to move out and in with your inhalation and exhalation. Let your eyes close to focus your inner awareness.

3. Choose one of the needs or desires and, focusing on your right hand, imagine you're holding its essence in your right palm. What does this need or desire look like? See its shape, color, degree of gloss. What does this need or desire feel like? Feel its weight, density, texture, temperature, degree of stillness. What does this need or desire sound like? Listen for its music, its voice. Thoroughly immerse yourself in the sights, sensations, and sounds of this need or desire.

4. When you're ready, shift your attention into your left palm. Imagine your left hand is holding the essence of the need or desire that seems to conflict with the one you just addressed. Repeat the process from step 3.

5. Now shift your awareness so that you can see and feel both hands, and what they each contain, at once. Still breathing deeply, letting your belly move with your breath, slowly lift your hands from your knees. Gradually bring your hands toward each other, watching and feeling the images and sensations in both hands.

6. Very slowly and gradually, bring your palms together so that their surfaces come entirely into contact with each other. Continue to breathe deeply and relax as you wait and watch, without expectation or demand, for whatever new images and sensations emerge. (If no new image emerges immediately, that's fine; it may become apparent to you in the next few days, perhaps when you least expect it.)

7. With your palms in firm contact with each other, rotate your hands to bring your thumbs to your chest, your fingers pointing upward. Bring any new images and sensations that

have emerged into your heart of compassion, surrounding them with your love.

8. With your palms still in firm contact with each other, rotate your hands to point your fingers downward. Bring the heels of your hands to your belly center, the point about two inches below your navel. Bring any new images and sensations that have emerged into your belly — your heart of creation — and infuse them with your pro-creative power.

9. Rest, absorbing and appreciating your experience of uniting polar opposites into a greater whole.

THE POWER OF BEING PRESENT

The cross-in-circle motif, also known as the World Cross, appears within prehistoric rock paintings and, in the historic era, within Celtic crosses.

In many cultures — not only in Northern European but also, for example, in African, Australian, and Indian traditions — the cross-in-circle represents the joining of male and female energies within one whole. The symbol demonstrates the totality encompassing complementary forces.

Your power to promote creation is the power of being present. Rather than living at the periphery of your life, you place yourself at the center of your world. Rather than being selfish, you are self-full.

Living at the center of your world, you recognize that others are living at the center of theirs, and you allow them their own

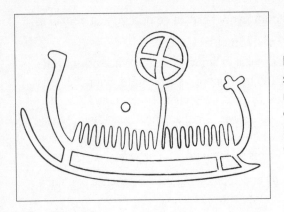

Rock carving shows a ship of regeneration bearing a cross-in-circle. Bottna, Bohuslän, Sweden, c. 3000–1000 B.C.E.

autonomy and self-determination. There's no need to control, fix, or change others. There's no need to attempt to manipulate others. There's no need to seek others' approval or validation. You're already home, free.

One day many years ago, I returned from a week's vacation and entered a gathering of co-workers in a large meeting hall. I had spent the week camping on my own, backpacking through the woods on steep mountain trails, sleeping in the open, carrying my own food and water. When I entered the hall, I saw each person surrounded by a soft glow; each person appeared to be an individual planet of light.

The vision was brief. But what made this way of seeing possible for even a moment? My recent experience of being so self-sufficient enabled me to see these people, at least for a moment, without expectation or need.

Dwelling in the experience of each moment, you're fully immersed in the mysterious, miraculous gift of being alive. How do you support yourself in being present? How do you return, again and again, to live in the center of your life?

The following Alignment exercise draws on the inspiration of Barbara Ann Brennan's *Light Emerging: The Journey of Personal Healing* as well as on the work of other writers and movement artists.[1] As you stand in and breathe through this Alignment exercise, feel the center of your body to be congruent with the center of the universe, the circle of life that surrounds you. Even as you focus on extending through the vertical dimension to connect with the universal spirit above and the earth's center below, feel as well the horizontal dimension that your elbows imply as they point out to each side. Feel yourself actively engaged in the expansion of your awareness. At the same time, you are at rest within the universe.

ALIGNMENT

Hold each position for ten or more cycles of the Centering Breath.

1. Taking a wide stance, place your feet two to three feet apart. Point your toes outward at a comfortable angle. Keeping your knees unlocked and slightly bent, position them directly over your toes.

2. Focus your gaze straight forward. Place your palms together at your belly center, your fingers pointing down toward the center of the earth.

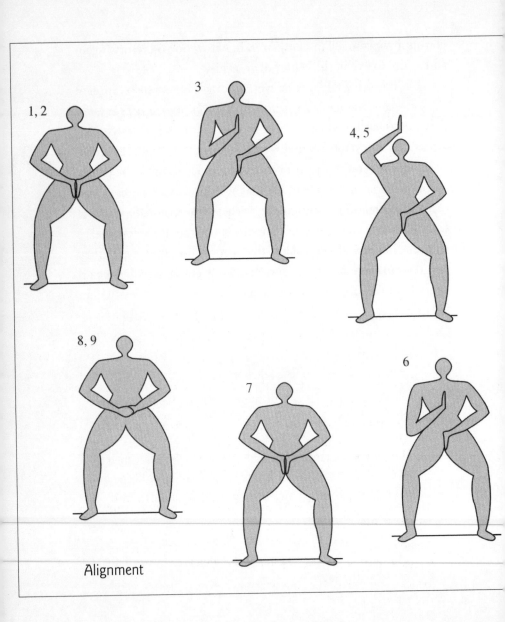

1, 2

3

4, 5

8, 9

7

6

Alignment

3. With your left hand remaining at your belly, raise your right hand up the midline of your body to the level of your heart, now pointing your fingers up toward the sky.

4. Raise your right hand farther up the midline of your body, coming to rest a few inches above the crown of your head, your fingers pointing upward.

5. See and feel a line of energy extending from your belly center down into the earth's center and at the same time reaching up through your heart, continuing up to and through the point where your individual spirit meets the universal spirit. Feel that you are aligning your belly's power to promote creation with your heart's desire and with the grace of heaven and earth.

6. Bring your right hand down to rest at the level of your heart.

7. Lower your right hand to bring your palms together again at your belly center, your fingers pointing down toward the center of the earth.

8. Come to stillness, releasing your hands to rest your palms over your belly center. Notice and feel any images and sensations occurring in your body.

9. Gradually return your awareness to this time and place.

Breath and image: Applying the Centering Breath, see and feel the line of energy stretching through your body's core, extending farther into earth and sky with each inhalation and releasing slightly with each exhalation. As you stand, breathing fully and deeply, feel your body's center congruent with the center of concentric spheres radiating outward expanding to the infinity of the universe.

Words of affirmation:

May all my actions be effortless;
may my heart's desires be manifest;
and may the universe accomplish her purpose through
*   me.*

Blessed be.

Part Three

Living a *Gutsy* Life

Chapter Thirteen

Designing Your Practice

Now that you've learned the core practices, the Energizing Breath, the warm-up/warm-down exercises, and the individual belly-energizing moves, you're ready to practice the sequence of moves as The Gutsy Women's Workout.

When and how often will you do the workout? Practicing it on a regular basis — investing ten minutes three times a week, or even five or six times a week — enables you to activate your soul power on a regular basis.

Repetition is what brings you the long-term benefits. With repetition, the movements become familiar to you and natural to your body, allowing you to focus more and more of your attention on living from your center.

The effects are cumulative. Today's practice builds on what you did yesterday and paves the way for what you'll do tomorrow. The benefits you receive in terms of vitality, pleasure, confidence, compassion, creativity, intuition, and sense of purpose are remarkable.

You might think that practicing a movement program on a regular basis requires discipline, which is no fun at all. But The Gutsy Women's Workout is not your usual exercise routine. You can create a belly-energizing practice that's so much fun — so affirming, so nurturing, so pleasurable — that you won't want to miss it. The trick is to personalize your program, keep renewing your motivation, record the benefits you receive, and conspire with friends.

> I practice the workout five or six days a week. It's a big part of my personal growth. Phenomenal things have happened. I feel my strength as a woman. In dance class I feel openness and strength coming from my belly. Being physically centered in myself is a powerful experience; I feel connected.
>
> — Mimi

PERSONALIZE YOUR PROGRAM

Timing is everything. What would be the best time for your practice? Some women like to practice in the morning to energize themselves and prepare for the day. Some rise early enough to practice before other members of the family awaken. One woman practices every morning in the minutes between when she turns on the coffeemaker and when the coffee is ready. Other women like to do the movement program after work or in the evening, before bed. They appreciate how the practice releases tension accumulated during the day and prepares them for restful sleep.

> I do the belly exercises in the morning before my kids wake up, and then I am in a good space for mothering for the rest of the day.
>
> — Sue

You may need to experiment to find the time that works for you. Whatever time you choose, treat it as an important commitment you have made to yourself. One woman, for example, writes her practice session onto her calendar — she's making an appointment to meet her Self, her very best friend.

When she first started her practice, another woman would set her alarm to wake her up thirty minutes earlier than usual. She'd get up and do her belly-energizing moves, and then follow her regular morning routine and go off to work on schedule. But as the days progressed, somehow the morning's supply of time expanded. She found that she could wake up at the usual time and, without that extra thirty minutes, do her morning practice and still be off to work on time.

> When I began practicing the belly-energizing exercises, I also began taking bold steps to move my career forward in ways I had never done before. I suddenly felt an inner strength and confidence in asking for what I want and need.
>
> — *Laura*

Once you learn the three warm-ups/warm-downs and the seven belly-energizing exercises, you can do the entire sequence in as little as five to seven minutes, which allows for a few repetitions of each movement. In order to receive more of its benefits, however, I suggest that you take ten or twenty minutes to practice the sequence when you can.

The length of your practice session depends on how many times you repeat each of the belly-energizing exercises and how fast you move through them. You can also complement your belly-energizing moves by doing one or more of the exercises for deepening awareness.

A deluxe practice session might include these elements, for example:

1. Naming Your Feelings

2. Setting Your Intention

3. Locating Your Center

4. Centering Breath (or another belly-breathing pattern of your choosing)

5. Awareness exercise: Draw Out Your Deepest Knowing

6. Warm-up exercises

7. The belly-energizing moves:

   - Bright Blessings

   - Belly Bowl

   - Power Centering

   - Lily

   - Wings

   - Tree

   - Alignment

8. Warm-down exercises

9. Awareness exercise: Draw Out Your Deepest Knowing

10. Awareness exercise: Dialogue with Your Inner Wisdom

11. Full-Body Breathing

Doing two rounds of the awareness exercise called Draw Out Your Deepest Knowing gives you before-and-after pictures of your belly's energy. The drawings give you visual evidence of the effect that the belly-energizing practice has on your body and mind.

You'll get the most benefit if you learn and practice the sequence of belly-energizing exercises in the order in which they're presented in this book. But practicing some of the belly-energizing moves is better than doing none at all. If you won't be practicing the whole sequence, pick and choose the moves you like best, making sure that your body is adequately prepared to practice them safely. If you begin with your favorite exercises, over time you may find yourself wanting to include additional moves in your repertoire.

Set the Stage

What would make your place for practicing the workout absolutely beautiful? What would you see, hear, touch, and smell there that would make you eager to be in that place?

Imagine the objects you'd like to see. Would there be inspiring words? What music, if any, would be playing? Would there be a scent of lavender or pine, or some other fragrance that invites you to breathe all the more deeply? Sight, sound, texture, scent — what about taste? If you practice in the morning, you can look forward to how good your breakfast will taste once you complete your session!

You'll find that doing the moves outdoors is a delight. Discover the sensation of practicing the belly-energizing exercises on a hilltop at sunrise, in the morning by a rushing mountain stream, in a pine forest on a sunny afternoon, or in the evening under the stars. Or how about doing the moves by a waterfall, on the beach, in a grove of oaks, in a garden of sunflowers, on the rim of a canyon, or in the center of an ancient circle of stones?

Make your place of practice not only beautiful but also convenient. You can copy the sequence of warm-ups/warm-downs and belly-energizing exercises in appendix 2 and post the illustrations on the wall at eye level next to the image of your intention. Then you won't have to guess which move comes next.

Accessorize

Consider the items you can use to access — that is, accessorize — your practice: clothing, fragrance, music, a recorded narration.

Clothing

Wear loose, comfortable tops and pants, clothes that allow you to move without restriction. Make sure your waistbands are loose and stretchable, giving you room to breathe.

Treat yourself to a special outfit, apparel you wear only for practice and for no other activity. When you put these garments on, you know that it's time to begin your practice and that this time is special. When you complete your session, change your clothes.

Allow yourself some extravagance. Practicing the program on a regular basis can guide you to the "pearl of great price" that is your center of being. If wearing a certain outfit inspires you to practice regularly, it's a bargain.

You might, in fact, give yourself two or three different outfits from which to choose. Then the question is not "Do I want to practice today?" but rather "Which outfit shall I wear when I practice today?"

You can lay out your special clothes in advance of your practice time. If your intention is to practice in the morning, for example, lay your outfit out the night before.

Fragrance

Dab your favorite perfume or essential oil on your wrist, inhaling the scent deeply as you begin your practice. Then, if you're ever feeling uncertain about doing the moves when the appointed time arrives, you can dab that same fragrance on your wrist, take a whiff, and you'll be moving and breathing without delay.

Music

Many women enjoy practicing the program in silence. They find that silence deepens their focus and increases their concentration, enhancing their receptivity to inner guidance. Others prefer to practice the program with musical accompaniment. If you always do the moves to the same music, putting that music on will cue you to begin the sequence. Then as your practice becomes established, you may enjoy moving to different styles of music to suit your mood. (See the resources at the end of the book for some musical suggestions.)

Narration

Record the following affirmations — or create your own declarations — and embody them as you practice the belly-energizing moves. This passage is an excerpt adapted from my book *Rite for Reconsecrating Our Womanhood*. (See the resources at the end of this book for more information.)

Bright Blessings: We ask for and receive the blessings of the earth, the trees, the sky, and we enter these blessings into our body's center.

Belly Bowl: Cherishing the bowl within our bellies, we trace the four directions — forward and back, north and south . . . and side to side, east and west. Rolling this bowl around its rim, in one direction and then the other, we encircle the creative power our bellies contain.

Power Centering: Alive within an ocean of energy, we reach out; we take and enter the power of creation into our body's center.

Lily: Descending into communion with ourselves and the earth, we replenish ourselves. Restored, we rise into relationship with others, heartfully, with open arms.

Wings: Securely supported by the earth and soaring into sky, we express the truth of who we are.

Tree: Rooted in the earth, reaching to sky, we acknowledge ourselves as kin to the trees.

Alignment: May all our actions be effortless. May our heart's desires be manifest. And may the universe accomplish her purpose through us. Blessed be.

KEEP RENEWING YOUR MOTIVATION

Sustaining a regular practice means continually renewing your interest and motivation. The following pointers suggest some ways you can keep yourself engaged in honoring and energizing your belly.

Give Yourself Reasons to Practice

When we give ourselves enough reasons, we can do just about anything. List and periodically update your reasons for practicing the belly-energizing program. What are the benefits you want to receive? What are the problems you want to eliminate?

One good reason to practice the program is to awaken the Source Energy that leads you into the experience of joy. As you live more and more through your center of being, you tap more deeply into your central joy, whatever that is for you.

YOUR CENTRAL JOY

What is your central joy? Make a sketch of concentric circles and then consider the following questions:

1. What is central to your joy? What is pivotal to your well-being? In the center of the concentric circles, write a word or phrase, or draw an image, describing this essential value.

2. What are the desires, relationships, thoughts, attitudes, activities, or events that take you away from your central joy? Somewhere on the chart, write a word or phrase, or draw an image, for each of these items. Draw a circle around each with an arrow pointing away from the center.

3. What are the desires, relationships, thoughts, attitudes, activities, or events that move you toward your central joy? Somewhere on the chart, write a word or phrase, or draw an image, for each of these items. Draw a circle around each with an arrow pointing toward the center.

4. How does practicing the belly-energizing exercises relate to your joy in life? Somewhere on the chart, write a word or phrase, or draw an image, for your belly-energizing practice. Draw a circle around it with an arrow indicating its relationship to your central joy.

However you name it, your greatest joy is waiting for you at your center of being. When you practice the belly-energizing exercises on a regular basis, you equip yourself to move into your center of being and take regular delight in your central joy.

Know Your Motivational Style

When you know what moves you into action, you can effectively support yourself in doing what you want to do. Knowing your motivational style, you can present the belly-energizing practice to yourself in a way that encourages you to stay with it.

HOW DO YOU MOTIVATE YOURSELF?

Remember a time when you started doing something new and kept on doing it. The activity could be anything — for example, driving a new way to work, taking up a sport, dining at a particular restaurant, or shopping at a certain store.

What provoked you to start this new activity and repeat it on a regular basis? Jot down your responses to these questions:

- Were you avoiding something you didn't want, or were you seeking something you did want?

- Were you doing it out of necessity, because you had to, or were you doing it because the option was available to you?

- Was it important to you that other people were doing it, too, or were you doing it regardless of what other people were doing?

- Was it important to you that other people would benefit from your action, or were you doing it entirely for your own benefit?

There are no right or wrong answers to these questions. Your answers simply indicate the ways in which you inspire yourself to act.

Now jot down your responses to these questions:

- What will practicing the belly-energizing moves help you to get?

- What will practicing the program help you to avoid or eliminate?

- In what way is practicing the belly-energizing program a necessity?

- How does practicing the moves open up new and exciting possibilities?

- Do you know you'll be joining many other women who are already practicing the belly-energizing sequence?

- Do you realize that when you practice the sequence you're doing something quite unique with respect to women's health and fitness?

- How will practicing the belly-energizing moves increase your own well-being?

- How will practicing the moves benefit your family, friends, co-workers, students, and clients?

The motives that get you started with the program may be different from the motives that keep you practicing it. For example, when I created this program, I really thought I had no choice: I had to do this or die. I didn't care what anyone thought of me or who else might benefit.

My motivation for continuing the practice is different. Now it's the experience of vitality and creativity, the possibilities for personal growth, the extraordinary people I meet, and the benefits I can share with others that keep me practicing this program. My motivation has largely shifted from necessity to possibility, from avoiding to seeking, and from personal well-being to shared interest.

Necessity and avoidance still play their part, though. I've done the practice long enough to know how wonderful I feel and how well the day goes when I've taken ten or fifteen minutes in the morning to energize my belly. I've come to expect this standard of well-being in the quality of my life. I want to avoid the dull and disorganized way I feel if I miss it. Consequently, I do the practice partly out of necessity — it's necessary for maintaining the good feelings I've come to expect.

Vary Your Program

Introduce novelty into your practice by combining the belly-energizing moves with journal writing, drawing, self-massage, or any of the breathing patterns. Experiment with the exercises for deepening awareness to make your program an enticing adventure.

Bypass Resistance

Sometimes you might feel resistance to practicing the moves. The following are some ways you can encourage yourself to keep energizing your belly.

Become an Investigator

If you find yourself resisting your practice, rather than judging or criticizing or coercing yourself, become an investigator, the detective on the case. As an objective yet caring observer, note exactly what you're thinking and how you're feeling; detail the particulars of your resistance.

What feelings do you witness? If you're feeling anxious, inquire gently — anxiety is often a fear of feeling. Perhaps you're feeling numb, grouchy, grumpy, bored, cranky, frightened, sluggish, resentful, depressed, restless, angry, or gloomy.

What thoughts do you witness? Resistance to doing your practice can show up with thoughts like "I'm too busy," "I don't have time," "It's too complicated," or "I don't have the energy for it." Those thoughts are usually excuses, because you always have time and energy to do what you want to do. What's underneath those excuses is usually some sort of fear — fear of being authentic, taking charge of your life, coming home to yourself.

Refuse to Cooperate with Oppression

We live in a culture that rewards women for taking care of others' needs, for playing out various kinds of addictions, and for being marketplace consumers. We live in a culture that characterizes women as inferior, subordinate, dangerous, exploitable. To the extent that we've internalized those oppressive images of who we are, we may fear challenging, releasing, and replacing them by discovering and expressing our own identity. At the same time, discovering and expressing our true nature is what we crave.

When I'm resisting my practice, what's usually stopping me is some form of internalized oppression. Once I recognize that, I ask myself, Do I love cooperating with and reinforcing the culture's oppression more than I love my life? Once I remember to ask the question, the answer is obvious, and I'm moving and breathing without a second thought.

Stage an Experiment

As the objective yet caring observer, you've noted your thoughts and feelings without judging or criticizing yourself. Now conduct an experiment, simply for the sake of gathering information. Investigate: will energizing your belly with movement and breath make any difference in the way you're thinking and feeling?

Do Just a Little

If you're feeling resistant, tell yourself you'll do just a few of the moves or just a few minutes of your practice. Promise yourself you can stop then, if you want to.

Some mornings, for example, I've stumbled out of bed grumbling and gloomy. On those mornings, I've said to myself, "I'll just do the first three moves. Nothing could make me feel worse than the way I'm feeling now."

By the time I've completed the third exercise, the gloom is beginning to lift. "I'll do just another two exercises," I say to myself, "and then I'll quit." So I do those moves, but then I don't want to stop. I'm actually beginning to feel rather perky. Before I know it, I've completed the sequence, ten or twenty minutes have gone by, and I'm ready to meet the day with a cheerful spirit. I remember, dimly, how horrible I felt only a few minutes earlier, and I'm grateful for the transformation that I've experienced in such a short time.

Give Yourself Permission to Do Nothing at All

In addition to the inner urge that declares, "I want to do this practice," there's often another opinion: "You *should* do this practice."

If you're feeling resistant, perhaps you're objecting not to the practice itself but rather to the idea that you "should" be doing it. When you graciously allow yourself to do nothing at all, you override the imperative that's getting in the way. The voice demanding "You should" fades away; the voice that says "I want to" now sings out clearly.

Refuse to Let Yourself Practice

There's often a third voice in the mix, an expression of internalized oppression that warns, "I won't let you! Don't you dare!" When you deliberately refuse to let yourself practice, then you're giving yourself the opportunity to resist your resistance. Pretty soon you may be saying, "I'm not allowed to do this? Oh, yeah? Just watch me!"

Resume Your Practice After a Break

If you miss some days, the following are some ways you can resume your practice without guilt or delay.

Gather the Data

Use any day that you miss doing your practice as a great opportunity to gather data on the effects of not doing the belly-energizing exercises. Having collected this information, you can perceive the benefits of energizing your belly all the more clearly.

Identify Yourself as a Regular Practitioner

Energizing your belly doesn't have to be an all-or-nothing proposition. If you miss some days of your practice, so what? Draw your attention to today, to this moment. Consider yourself someone who does the practice on a regular basis; you get to define what "regular" means to you. Tell yourself, "I'm a person who does my practice regularly," and notice how that's already the case.

GATHER SUPPORT

If you live in a household with family or friends, determine what kind of support you'd like from them for practicing your program, and ask for it. Let those who depend on you know that you'll need a certain amount of uninterrupted time on certain days. Negotiate ways in which the other members of the household can cooperate in making this time available for you.

Let these people know, too, that by supporting you in taking this time for yourself, they're serving their own interests as well as yours. As you renew and revitalize yourself with your belly-energizing practice, you'll be able to attend to their needs with all the more patience and pleasure.

And congratulate yourself for setting a good example. By taking time to honor and energize your belly, you're demonstrating a practical way to move beyond dependence, deepening into the source of nurturing that abides within each of us. As one woman says, "My family loves it when I take care of myself this way. It spills over into everyone recognizing what they are able to do, taking more responsibility for themselves, enjoying more freedom."

This morning I didn't do my usual belly-energizing practice. During the rest of the day, I kept feeling as if I were missing something. Tonight, as I was staring at the ceiling wondering why my day felt so flat, I unconsciously started to breathe into my belly. Suddenly, the breathing became more conscious, and I increased the breath. I felt more alive, and contained more energy than I had all day. It is a good lesson, one that I will bring with me into each day.

— Tricia

Tell People about Your Experience

As you practice your belly-energizing program, you may want to share with others the insights and benefits you experience. Speak about your experience to people who will be supportive rather than skeptical. You can face the critics and naysayers later. At the beginning, though, when you're exploring what honoring your belly means to you, treat yourself to all the encouragement you deserve. One woman told me, "My friend saw me doing the exercises when I was camping, and she said, 'Looks great!' "

Conspire with Friends

When you share your experience with other women, they may want to join you in practicing the belly-energizing moves. That's great; you'll have good company on your adventure, and you'll have lots of fun together.

> After a busy day at work it was such a comfort and treat to get together and exercise as a group. It was wonder-full. I felt so much energy. The charge we created — *wow!* I feel inspired to practice more.
>
> — *Patty*

When you do the workout in a circle of women, you're literally "conspiring" — that is, *breathing together*. Doing the belly-energizing exercises in the company of other women generates extraordinary energy.

If you're inspired to convene a circle of women for learning and doing the practice together, consider the following suggestions to complement your organizational know-how. Invite some friends to get together with you to explore the possibilities. Since bellies are such a tender subject for most women, at the first meeting pay special attention to creating a comfortable setting, one that encourages mutual respect and leaves no room for fault-finding, blame, or criticism.

Begin by describing your own interest in honoring your body's center, and then invite each of the other women to speak about her interest. Ask the group to allow each woman to speak without interruption for a few minutes. Ask each woman to complete her comments within a certain time frame so that everyone present has a chance to speak. You might also guide the women in doing the Centering Breath and one of the exercises for deepening awareness. Provide an opportunity for each woman to share her response to these experiences as the others listen attentively. In this way, the women will get to know and trust one another.

At the end of this gathering, if there's interest in continuing to meet, find a date, time, and place that's convenient for all concerned. You might want to get together on a weekly basis, or you might want to schedule a weekend getaway.

Even if your group initially numbers just two — you and one other woman — that's great! As others see and hear about the effect of the practice on your two lives, interest will grow.

As the group practice evolves, invite everyone to participate in making the place of practice as welcoming and comfortable as possible. Likewise, invite everyone to participate in designing the flow of activities that take place during your time together.

> Being in a circle of women I know and love, having time together to learn a practice to honor ourselves, I experience them and myself in many new ways.
>
> — Sue

A gathering might begin with one or more of the core practices — for example, with the Centering Breath. Then each woman might take some time to check in, saying how she is feeling in the moment, how her week has been, how she has been experiencing her belly power. Following these "belly stories," you might review and practice the moves you've already learned, and then go on to learn one or two new exercises. You might then do one of the exercises for deepening awareness. Your session could conclude with Full-Body Breathing.

Depending on the amount of time you have together, follow your practice with a potluck dinner or singing, drumming, and telling bawdy jokes in the grand tradition of Baubo, the belly goddess.

LETTER FROM THE FUTURE

Imagine that you've already created and integrated a powerful, pleasurable belly-energizing practice into your life. From a vantage point in the future, write a letter to a friend. Date it six months or a year from now and describe the following:

- Now that you've made a regular time and place for energizing your belly, what's your life like? What changes have taken place?

- What keeps you practicing your belly-energizing moves on a regular basis? What benefits are you receiving?

- What time and place have you chosen for your practice?

- What do you see, smell, hear, touch, taste, and feel during this time and in this place that makes doing the practice safe, nurturing, and totally irresistible?

- What might have detoured you from practicing regularly? How have you bypassed those detours?

- What has supported you in practicing regularly? How have you gathered this support?

ANY PLACE, ANY TIME

Beyond practicing The Gutsy Women's Workout at your regular time and place, how can you kindle your pro-creative power in various moments and settings throughout your day?

The Centering Breath and the other breathing patterns are certainly portable. You'll be breathing anyway as you're on the job, driving through traffic, waiting for a health care appointment, shopping, cooking, cleaning, washing the dishes, doing the laundry, and the rest. You can always choose to breathe in a way that refreshes you.

Practicing the Perineal Squeeze is an option at many times during the day — for example, when you're in the car and stopped at a red light. (I can only imagine women across the nation, across the world, grinning to ourselves as we practice the Perineal Squeeze at roadway intersections. We'd be giving new meaning to the term "red-light district.")

If you're feeling stressed at work, you can, as some women do, go into the bathroom and do a few rounds of the Energizing Breath. If you're hiking up a steep hill, use Power Centering to propel yourself up the slope.

You can use some of the belly-energizing exercises, or the entire sequence, as a preparation for any sport or movement practice. Incorporating these *hara*-charging moves into your yoga, tai chi, qigong, or dance flow will make your experience all the more delicious; being more centered, you'll reduce the possibility of injuring yourself as well.

The belly-energizing moves and breath patterns also make an excellent prelude to any artistic endeavor. As one woman, a songwriter, says, "The workout's a great way to start a creative process because you get so much energy from it."

Do you meet with a group of women on a regular basis? When they hear about the workout's benefits from you, they may want to incorporate the practice as part of the group's ongoing agenda.

Once you're familiar with the Alignment exercise and feel comfortable sharing it with others, you might introduce this practice and its significance to a group of your co-workers. Invite people to stand in a circle and lead them into the Centering Breath. Then guide them through the gestures that comprise the Alignment exercise as you explain their meaning. Practicing Alignment with your co-workers supports each person in applying creativity and confidence to her intention. At the same time, it brings each individual's intention into cooperative relationship with others' intentions and with the group's purpose as a whole. Imagine working in a setting in which people's intentions support one another seamlessly!

RECORD THE BENEFITS YOU RECEIVE

Keeping a journal is one of the most powerful tools you can use to create and maintain a regular practice. You can use your journal to record your responses to the exercises for deepening awareness. You can also use it to record the benefits you receive from each move and from the practice as a whole, together with the insights and intuitions emerging during your practice sessions. You can use it to note whether you choose to practice on any given day and the effect of your choice.

A mother with three preteen daughters kept a journal of her belly-energizing practice and her life over a seven-month period. In her journal she noted whether she practiced in the morning, afternoon, or evening and whether the pace of her practice was slow, moderate, or fast. The following are four of her entries:

> After doing the moves I felt very centered — even under a lot of stress at work, I was able to stay calm and focused. I look forward to doing the moves again tomorrow....

> I did my moves before an audience this morning. Two of my daughters watched; then one of them stood behind me and began following along!...

> My resistance choice was to start the day with an early morning walk. The feeling of centeredness and the ability to focus was not as prominent as yesterday....

> It felt so good to do the moves after skipping one day! I felt great through the day — boundless energy — big accomplishments.

You can use your journal to lay the foundation for the next day's practice. When you complete your entry for one day, skip a few lines or turn to a new page and write the next day's date. The journal is now primed to receive your next entry.

SAMPLE JOURNAL PAGE

Today's date: _____

Time of day I practiced: _____

The moves I did: _____

What inspired me to begin: _____

_____

How I felt before practicing: _____

_____

How I felt after practicing: _____

_____

Moves I especially enjoyed: _____

_____

Benefits I received: _____

_____

Images, insights, and affirmations: _____

_____

What I noticed about my breath and belly during the day:

_____

Other reflections: _____

_____

CHECKLIST: DESIGNING YOUR PRACTICE

◉ Create a consistent time for your practice.

◉ Choose special clothes to wear.

◉ Create a beautiful, healthy, and inspiring environment:

- ◆ Establish a place to display whatever words, images, and objects please you.

- ◆ Place your image of intention on the wall at eye level, to serve as your visual focus as you do the moves and to help you direct the energy that you are activating.

- ◆ Enhance your space with a favorite fragrance.

- ◆ Play your favorite music — make your own mix of selections from a variety of albums. Or, keep several types of music on hand to suit a variety of moods — exuberant, contemplative, soulful, or spunky.

◉ Keep your journal, blank paper, and crayons or colored markers nearby to record the insights, guidance, affirmations, and inspiration that emerge as you practice.

Chapter Fourteen

Restoring Your World

Now you have what it takes to practice The Gutsy Women's Workout in a way that fits into your day and your life. What difference will it make? What difference will having more vitality, pleasure, confidence, compassion, creativity, intuition, and sense of purpose make in the everyday details of your life?

More vitality means your life force is flowing more fully and freely — the definition of health and healing. With more vitality, you're more receptive to and savvy about sensual and sexual pleasure. You're all the more equipped to share such pleasures in intimate relationships with others.

Nourished by vitality and pleasure, you have the confidence to be with family, friends, and co-workers in relationships of mutual respect. Your heart full to overflowing, you can be patient, generous, and compassionate with them while still attending to your own well-being.

Confidence and compassion enable you to speak up and out, to express what you know to be true. Expressing your originality, you also draw on your intuition, coming up with creative ways to solve problems and introduce innovations at home, at work, and in your community.

Vitality, pleasure, confidence, compassion, creativity, intuition, and sense of purpose — all are qualities and capacities that support you in clarifying your heart's desire and actually living in alignment with your soul's purpose. When you're living in such alignment, you're not just following your bliss — you're living your bliss.

Bliss. That's the bonus of living a gutsy life. That's the bonus for honoring your belly and energizing the soul power concentrated in your body's center.

Taking charge of your pro-creative power, coming home to yourself, puts you at the center of your world. And rather than being self-absorbed, you're self-fulfilled. The experience of self-fulfillment allows you to sense your kinship with creation.

The exercises had a surprising effect in my life. I found myself feeling more empowered and more "myself." I began to confidently pursue things that had previously caused me great anxiety. Opportunities began to arise and gave me the chance to review what I really wanted. I found that I needed to realign my intention. Without the sense of empowerment I received from the exercises, I would still be stuck, depressed, and lacking focus. Now I am focused, clear about my intention, confident, and taking action steps to achieve my dreams.

— *Anna*

Your sense of kinship with creation affirms your intimate connection with the web of life. You know, in your gut, that what happens to another creature is also happening to you. It's not just that redwood tree that's being logged for decks on second homes; it's not just that river that's being trashed by a factory's waste stream; it's not just that sky that's being clouded by weather-modifying chemicals. It's your tree, your river, your sky. Their fate is not separate from yours. A question then arises: What's your responsibility for protecting them?

> As I opened my eyes after the Alignment exercise, I found myself looking out through the picture window and saw the fir tree out there. My fingers were the tree's fingers. The tree's light green needles at the tips of its branches were like fingers, like my fingers.
>
> — *Elaine*

Honoring and activating your *hara* power doesn't necessarily mean you'll be walking the picket lines, carrying placards, or camping outside the president's door. If that's your choice, firing up your *hara* power will certainly help give you the guts to do so. But it's not required.

Simply by being who you are — setting the example of a self-validating woman living in alignment with her soul purpose — you're being the change this world needs if we humans are to survive.

IN GAIA'S LAP

What are the dimensions of the ecological crisis occurring across this planet? Scientists predict that we'll make the planet uninhabitable in the foreseeable future. According to Deep Ecology activist

John Seed, the rate of environmental destruction is so rapid that unless we spark "an unprecedented revolution in consciousness," no action that we take now can save us. "Nothing but a miracle would be of any use," he declares.[1]

I believe that women — you, me, all of us — can be that miracle. What do you imagine would happen if women acknowledged the pro-creative power we carry within our body's center? We would know indisputably, in our guts, that our bodies are the earth's body. What degrades the earth — the goddess Gaia, as the Greeks named her — damages us. What nourishes the earth nurtures us.

When we love our bellies, we open to a tender, intimate connection with the planet. As we allow ourselves to breathe deeply, we notice the quality of the air. As we allow ourselves to eat in peace, we notice the quality of our food and we care about the soil in which it grows. As we feel our kinship with the trees, we notice the fate of the forests.

We have been sitting in Gaia's lap for a long time. Now it's time for us to hold her in ours.

ALTERNATIVES TO OBSESSION

As we obsess about our body weight and shape, American women bankroll the cosmetic-surgery and weight-loss industries with more than $40 billion each year. What else could we do with our $40 billion?

What do you imagine would happen if instead of trying to banish our bellies, we directed our life force and our money to healing the distress within our communities, our nations, the world? What would happen if instead of trying to shrink our stomachs, we used the resources we already have to ensure humankind's survival? What do you imagine would happen if women took charge of our pro-creative power and claimed it as our own? We would discover that we already possess the courage, confidence, passion, compassion, creativity, and insight that we need in order to act on behalf of the earth and all her creatures.

For millennia, women have expressed our pro-creative power by bearing and raising healthy children. Our pro-creative power has always worked through us to ensure the survival of our lineage, our family, our tribe. The birth-giving capacity of our bellies has ensured the survival, and evolution, of the human species.

For nearly two years, my grandmother had been coming to me in my meditations. I knew she was bringing a gift for me, but for eighteen months I wouldn't even look at what she was holding. When I was willing to look at it, I saw that she was holding a gold ball of energy. After another few months, I took the ball from her and I brought it into my belly. After that, everything fell into place. A community development foundation asked me to be its director. I accepted the job once the board agreed to my plan for genuine grassroots empowerment.

— Linda

In these times, our tribe is all of life. Our home encompasses all of Earth. Today women have the opportunity — perhaps the calling — to apply our pro-creative power to preserving life on this planet.

Imagine: We cultivate and direct our pro-creative power to generate peace, justice, and ecological sustainability within every realm of human endeavor. Imagine: We bring our pro-creative power to bear as we establish new ways to feed, shelter, educate, employ, entertain, inspire, and govern ourselves. We organize new ways to promote our health, resolve our conflicts, serve one another, protect one another, and preserve the life of the natural world.

Where do we start? We start with ourselves. We value and validate ourselves. We celebrate our body's center as the chalice of our sacred wisdom and spiritual power.

OUR FUTURE, OUR CHOICE

Contemporary Western culture shames women's bellies, and it's a clever tactic. Shame makes a woman's belly an uncomfortable place to be.

To avoid feeling such discomfort, we're tempted to lose touch with the pro-creative power our bellies shelter, withdrawing our awareness and abandoning our body's center. If we do so, what's the result? Conveniently for the culture, we barely notice that our soul power is leaking away. Then we wonder why we feel so empty inside, gutted, harboring a hole that nothing can fill and a hunger that nothing can satisfy.

Many women, me included, have tried to flatten our bellies and hide them from sight. We hope that by removing the target we'll avoid the shame and the abuse. We try to comply with the culture's conventions. Like hostages becoming loyal to our captors, we cooperate with our own oppression.

But when we make our bellies rigid, we cut ourselves off from our core energy, our pro-creative power. We make our body's center the focus of our self-contempt. We unconsciously work the culture's violence upon ourselves.

The culture entices us to become agents for our own disempowerment. It urges us to enforce its restrictions on ourselves and one another — with diet pills and weight-loss plans, cosmetic surgery, stick-figured dress-up dolls, and instant-slimming undergarments.

The culture constantly bombards us with directives to belittle our bellies. But the good news is this:

We do not have to torture ourselves any longer.

We don't have to make the culture's cruelty our own. We don't have to enforce its oppression upon ourselves, our friends, our daughters, our sisters.

We can choose to cherish our body's center, our center of being. We can ungirdle our bellies and let ourselves breathe and feel. We can take charge and express the creative power that we already carry within us.

In class tonight, as we were doing the moves, I received a picture of how the energy was moving. It was like a stone dropping into a pond, producing oval ripples that radiated outward. With each breath, this energy increased, big waves of belly energy rippling throughout the room, passing on out of the building, on out through the whole city. Later, when we were doing the workout again, there was a point when we were all in sync, and all fully concentrating within. Here again, we were building up this pond effect. Each breath, each gesture, each woman was producing bigger and bigger ripples. Who knows? Maybe our belly energy rippled all the way east to the Atlantic, north to Canada, south to Florida, and west to the Pacific!

— Tricia

As we enliven our bellies, we can consider ourselves to be cultural pioneers. In every moment that we honor our bellies, we are revaluing and reconsecrating our womanhood. We are transforming our culture. We are creating a new world.

This is my prayer: May we know ourselves as sacred beings.

Women's Bellies
in History and Culture

When I first started this belly-energizing practice, I'd experience a vague sense of dread from time to time. You, too, may notice a subtle — or obvious — nagging feeling that you're doing something wrong. Nothing criminal, exactly, but nothing conventionally acceptable, either.

If at times you feel a bit uneasy as you cultivate the Source Energy within your belly, remember that you're reversing a trend Western culture has sustained for thousands of years: disempowering women by shaming our bellies and appropriating our procreative power. Your uneasiness may signal that you're tapping into a collective, cellular memory of the overt and covert violence that Western culture has worked against women's bellies.

Western culture has made women's bellies a target of assault.

As gruesome as the details are, acknowledging the scope of the violence helps to validate and ground whatever uncomfortable feelings may arise. The information gives your feelings context. It also reminds you of the courage you demonstrate in reclaiming your pro-creative power.

However gut-wrenching it is to learn about the culture's history of violence against women and our bellies, such learning is also liberating. We can realize that whatever shame we might feel with respect to our bellies, the shame isn't really ours — it's an artifact of our culture.

Do not use this information to cast yourself as a victim of cultural forces. As you read on, notice how you're breathing, and allow your breath to lengthen and deepen. Let this information provoke you to live and breathe all the more fully in the present, expressing the power to promote creation that's already within you.

OUR HISTORY, OUR CULTURE

For five thousand years, Western culture has attempted to commandeer the pro-creative power that we women shelter within our bellies. Our culture has defined our bellies as targets of assault, resources to exploit, and objects to control. The modern methods of disempowerment include incest and rape, assault on pregnant women, unnecessary hysterectomies and cesarean sections, restrictions on women's authority in pregnancy and childbirth, and inappropriate use of reproductive technology.

In our effort to avoid the culture's violence, many women — me included — have internalized its animosity. We've targeted our bellies and inflicted injury on ourselves. We've enforced the culture's oppression on ourselves.

In the context of our history and culture, honoring our bellies and activating our pro-creative power takes guts. With courage, and with compassion for ourselves and for one another, we can reclaim our pivotal power and direct it to serve our central purpose.

WOMEN'S BELLIES AS TARGETS OF ASSAULT

⊛ Although scholars' estimates vary, it's likely that at least eighty thousand women and perhaps two hundred and fifty thousand women or more were put to death or died in prison during the witch craze in fifteenth- through eighteenth-century Europe. Many of the women who were killed were midwives, herbalists, and healers — women who possessed the traditional knowledge and skills for sustaining women's pro-creative power.[1]

The executioners hung, burned, and tortured women. One method of torture was forcing water down a woman's throat, then beating on her bloated belly with paddles and sticks.[2]

⊛ A woman is raped in the United States every six minutes.[3]

Rape is used as a weapon of war. In the 1990s, for example, an estimated fifty thousand Bosnian women, ranging in age from six to seventy years old, were raped by enemy soldiers. During the 1994 genocide in Rwanda, as many as five hundred thousand women and girls were tortured and raped.[4]

❧ In the United States, at least 25 percent of pregnant teenagers are battered by their intimate partners before, during, or just after their pregnancy; some estimates are as high as 80 percent. Among pregnant women of all ages, as many as 37 percent experience violence at the hands of their intimate partners. Abuse frequently begins or intensifies during a woman's pregnancy.[5]

Murder is the leading cause of death among pregnant and recently pregnant women.[6]

❧ Hysterectomy is the second most common major surgery performed upon women of reproductive age in the United States. More than six hundred thousand hysterectomies are performed in the United States each year, costing more than $5 billion, as estimated in 1993.[7]

At least 70 percent of the hysterectomies performed in the United States are unnecessary.[8]

More than one-fourth of all American women will have had a hysterectomy by the age of sixty.[9]

❧ Cesarean section — surgical removal of a baby from a woman's uterus — is the most common major surgery performed upon women of reproductive age in the United States.[10]

In the United States, the rate of births by cesarean section has been steadily rising since 1996. In 2003, nearly 30 percent of births were by cesarean. The rate of cesarean deliveries has been increasing among all women, including women in their first pregnancies with healthy babies positioned correctly for birth.[11]

While cesarean sections can be lifesaving operations for both mothers and babies, unnecessary procedures more than triple the risk of death during childbirth and increase the risk of post-delivery infection.

WOMEN'S BELLIES AS RESOURCES TO EXPLOIT

◈ In the United States, from the nineteenth century through the first decades of the twentieth century, educating women to take charge of their procreative power was illegal.[12] Information about preventing conception — even about preventing venereal disease — was considered obscene. Providing such information was punishable by a thirty-year prison sentence.

◈ Nearly half of all pregnancies in the United States are accidental, including more than 30 percent of pregnancies occurring among married couples.[13]

Based on current abortion rates, one out of three American women will have had an abortion by the time she is forty-five years old.[14]

Before abortion was legalized in the United
States, an estimated five thousand women died
annually as a result of illegal abortions. The
legalization of abortion in the United States nearly
eliminated deaths due to the procedure.[15]

- Reproductive technology — including artificial
  insemination, embryo transfer, in vitro fertilization,
  the use of surrogate mothers, and cloning —
  industrializes the birth process, removing it from
  the context of women's bodies.[16]

  Reproductive technology may compensate for, and
  serve to mask, the increasing infertility among women
  and men corresponding to the prevalence of industrial
  pollutants and pathogens in our environment.[17]

WOMEN'S BELLIES AS OBJECTS TO CONTROL

- Samuel Johnson, one of eighteenth-century England's
  most influential figures, plainly stated the culture's
  envy of the power women hold within our bellies:
  "Nature has given women so much power that the
  law has very wisely given them little."[18]

- A Virginia law that was still on the books in 1990
  required a woman to wear a corset while dancing in
  public. If she danced without wearing a corset, or if
  she adjusted it while she was dancing, the authorities
  could shut down the dance hall.[19]

- The American Society for Aesthetic Plastic Surgery reports that one hundred and forty-five thousand tummy tucks were performed on women in 2004, a 30 percent increase from the previous year and nearly a 350 percent increase since 1997. At an average cost of $5,000 per tuck, women spent $725 million on tummy tucks in 2004.[20]

- Americans spend more than $40 billion on dieting and diet-related products each year.[21]

- Most fashion models are thinner than 98 percent of American women; 80 percent of American women are dissatisfied with their looks.[22]

- On any given day, 50 percent of American women are trying to lose weight, mainly by dieting.[23]

- By the time they are ten years old, 80 percent of American girls have started dieting.[24]

- As many as 8 percent of "normal dieters" will develop eating disorders.[25]

- In the United States, an estimated twenty-five million girls and women have eating disorders. Eating disorders are on the rise among women in midlife.[26]

  Anorexia is a leading cause of death among young women. Within ten years of the eating disorder's onset, 5 to 10 percent of anorexics die from related causes, including cardiac arrest and suicide.[27]

HONORING OUR BELLIES

Honoring our bellies is an act of cultural renewal. In every moment that we honor our bellies, we are revaluing ourselves and reconsecrating our womanhood. We are actively creating a world that affirms and cherishes life.

In these early days of the twenty-first century, reclaiming our body's center as sacred, not shameful, may seem unconventional. Still, as we persevere with our cultural pioneering, we can revel in the bliss of coming home to ourselves — and at the same time set the stage for humankind's survival.

The Gutsy Women's Workout

These pages display the illustrations for the three warm-up/ warm-down exercises and the seven belly-energizing exercises that comprise The Gutsy Women's Workout. Feel free to copy these illustrations and post them at eye level in the place where you'll be practicing the moves.

To ensure your safety and comfort, refer to chapter 5, Practice Pointers, for the full range of guidelines for practice, including the preparations and specific dos and don'ts.

As You Begin

Start with the core practices detailed in chapter 1 and:

- Give yourself room to breathe
- Locate your center

- Enter into the Centering Breath
- Name your feelings in this moment
- Affirm your intention

Then move on to the following:

- Prepare for vigorous movement with the three warm-up/warm-down exercises.
- Move slowly and smoothly. Attend to what you're doing.
- Move within your comfort zone; never strain, push, or force yourself.
- Ease out of vigorous movement with the three warm-up/warm-down exercises.

Enjoy!

The Gutsy Women's Workout
Warm-Up/Warm-Down Exercises

1 • Side Stretches • Centering Breath
3 repetitions each side

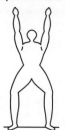 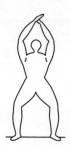 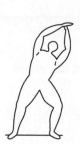 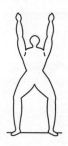 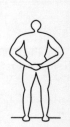

2 • Diagonal Stretches • Centering Breath
3 repetitions each side

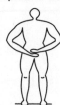 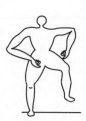 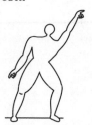 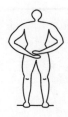 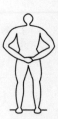

3 • Cradle • Centering Breath
5 repetitions

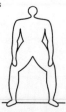 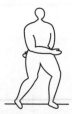 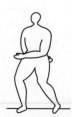 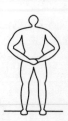

The Gutsy Women's Workout
Belly-Energizing Exercises

1 • VITALITY • Bright Blessings • Energizing Breath
5 repetitions

  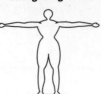 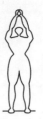 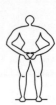

2 • PLEASURE • Belly Bowl • Centering Breath
5 repetitions forward and back, side-to-side, then circling in each direction

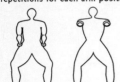   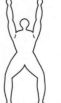 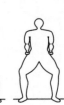

3 • CONFIDENCE • Power Centering • Energizing Breath
3 repetitions for each arm position

    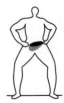

4 • COMPASSION • Lily • Energizing Breath
7 repetitions

 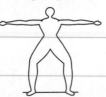 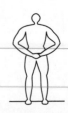

The Woman's Belly Book by Lisa Sarasohn (New World Library)
Copyright © 2006 Self-Health Education, Inc. • www.loveyourbelly.com

The Gutsy Women's Workout
Belly-Energizing Exercises

5 • CREATIVITY • Wings • Energizing Breath
3 repetitions each side

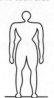 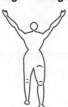 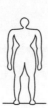 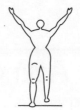 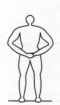

6 • INTUITION • Tree • Centering Breath
Hold each position for ten cycles of breath

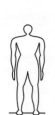 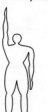 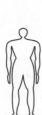 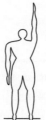 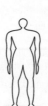 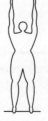 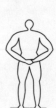

7 • PURPOSE • Alignment • Centering Breath
Hold each position for ten cycles of breath

 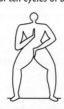 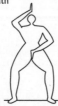 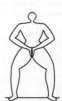 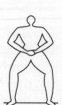

The Woman's Belly Book by Lisa Sarasohn (New World Library)
Copyright © 2006 Self-Health Education, Inc. • www.loveyourbelly.com

Acknowledgments

What amounts to a small nation of women and men has helped me to bring this book into being. I thank each and every one of you. You've inspired, challenged, instructed, aided, cheered, and encouraged me for years. You know who you are.

My thanks go to all the women who have sponsored my workshops. Together, we've created the opportunity for so many women to become belly-proud.

Each woman who has participated in my workshops and responded to my writing has been a shining source of inspiration. As we've shared our stories, we've become belly buddies, belly friends. Thank you.

I'm grateful to my family for their enduring support.

A shout goes out to local and New World librarians for their generous assistance and continuing encouragement.

The Unitarian Universalist Women's Federation supported the production of the related instructional video. Thank you.

I honor all the women who have held the red thread of women's wisdom through each generation, passing it on to the next.

And I thank the Muse in all her many guises.

Notes

Chapter 1: Core Principles, Core Practices

1. Clarissa Pinkola Estés, *Women Who Run With the Wolves: Myths and Stories of the Wild Woman Archetype* (New York: Ballantine, 1992), p. 13.

2. Anne Lamott, "Let Us Commence," *Salon*, June 6, 2003, http://www.salon.com/mwt/col/lamott/2003/06/06/commencement/index1.html (accessed December 2, 2005).

3. Dennis McCarty, email message to author, November 8, 2002; Rufus C. Camphausen, *The Yoni: Sacred Symbol of Female Creative Power* (Rochester, VT: Inner Traditions, 1996), pp. 2–3; Frank Waters, *Book of the Hopi* (New York: Penguin, 1977), pp. 10–11; Andrew Ellis and others, *Grasping the Wind* (Brookline, MA: Paradigm Publications, 1989), p. 309; and Kenneth S. Cohen, *The Way of Qigong: The Art and Science of Chinese Energy Healing* (New York: Ballantine Books, 1997), pp. 342–44.

4. Reverend Jeanette Stokes, personal communication with author, December 1997.

5. Eve Ensler, preface to *The Good Body* (New York: Villard/Random House, 2004).

Chapter 2: A Cultural Exposé

1. Anne Hollander, *Seeing Through Clothes* (New York: The Viking Press, 1978), pp. 97, 98, 110.

2. Naomi Wolf, *The Beauty Myth: How Images of Beauty Are Used Against Women* (New York: Anchor/Doubleday, 1992), p. 184.

3. Sara Kingdon, MD, telephone conversation with author, November 22, 1998.

4. Winifred Lubell, *The Metamorphosis of Baubo: Myths of Women's Sexual Energy* (Nashville, TN: Vanderbilt University Press, 1994), pp. 22–24.

5. Robert Lawlor, *Sacred Geometry: Philosophy and Practice* (London: Thames and Hudson, 1982), pp. 23–31.

6. *Encyclopedia of Religion* (New York: Macmillan, 1987), s. v. "Labyrinth" (by Lima De Freitas).

7. J. A. Simpson and E. S. C. Weiner, *Oxford English Dictionary*, 2nd ed. (Oxford: Clarendon Press, 1989), 19:519.

8. Barbara Walker, *The Woman's Dictionary of Symbols and Sacred Objects* (San Francisco: Harper and Row, 1988), pp. 160–61.

Chapter 3: What's In a Belly?

1. Kenneth S. Cohen, *The Way of Qigong: The Art and Science of Chinese Energy Healing* (New York: Ballantine Books, 1997), pp. 117–21.

2. Elinor Gadon, *The Once and Future Goddess: A Symbol for Our Time* (San Francisco: Harper and Row, 1989), p. 2.

3. *Belly Buttons: How Are You Still Connected to Your Mother?* VHS, produced and directed by Judith Selby (Forest Knolls, CA, 1993).

Chapter 4: Secrets of Your Body's Center

1. M. Babyak and others, "Exercise Treatment for Major Depression," *Psychosomatic Medicine* 62, no. 5 (September 2000), pp. 633–38.

2. Quoted in Harriet Brown, "The *Other* Brain Also Deals with Many Woes," Health and Fitness, *New York Times*, August 23, 2005. See also Yvette Taché, PhD, and Mulugeta Million, PhD, "Stress, Visceral Pain and the Brain-Gut Connections," in *Chronic Abdominal and Visceral Pain: Theory and Practice*, ed. P. J. Pasricha, W. D. Willis, and G. F. Gebhart (New York: Taylor and Francis, 2006).

3. Brown, "The *Other* Brain."

4. American Psychiatric Association, "307.50 Eating Disorder Not Otherwise Specified," in *Diagnostic and Statistical Manual of Mental Disorders*,

4th ed. (Washington, DC: American Psychiatric Association, 2000), http://www.poppink.com/dsmiv/14.html (accessed December 29, 2005).

5. See references cited in notes 22 through 26 for appendix 2 below.

6. Adapted from National Eating Disorders Association, "What's Going On with Me? Evaluating Eating and Exercise Habits," http://www.national eatingdisorders.org/p.asp?WebPage_ID=286&Profile_ID=41155 (accessed December 29, 2005); and Renfrew Center, "Do You Have a Healthy Relationship with Food?" http://www.renfrewcenter.com/interactive-quiz.asp (accessed December 29, 2005).

7. *Encyclopedia of Religion* (New York: Macmillan, 1987), s. v. "Breath and Breathing" (by Ellison Banks Findly).

8. Karlfried Graf von Dürckheim, "Hara in the Japanese Language," in *Hara: The Vital Centre of Man* (London: Unwin, 1984), pp. 47–61; Kiiko Matsumoto and Stephen Birch, *Hara Diagnosis: Reflections on the Sea* (Brookline, MA: Paradigm Publications, 1988), pp. 10–11; and Seigen Yamaoka, *The Art and the Way of Hara*, rev. ed. (Union City, CA: Heian International, 1992), pp. 4–5.

9. Joan Halifax, *Shaman Voices: A Survey of Visionary Narratives* (New York: E. P. Dutton, 1979), p. 55; and Richard Katz, *Boiling Energy: Community Healing Among the Kalahari Kung* (Cambridge, MA: Harvard University Press, 1982).

10. *Encyclopedia of Religion*, s. v. "Breath and Breathing."

11. Robert Lawlor, *Voices of the First Day: Awakening in the Aboriginal Dreamtime* (Rochester, VT: Inner Traditions, 1991), p. 372.

12. Frank Waters, *Book of the Hopi* (New York: Penguin, 1977), pp. 10–11.

13. Marilyn Youngbird, lecture presented at the School of Spiritual Healing, Black Mountain, NC, May 9–12, 1996.

14. Brooke Medicine Eagle, *Moon Time* (Polson, MT: 1987), audiotape of lecture.

15. Kenneth S. Cohen, *The Way of Qigong: The Art and Science of Chinese Energy Healing* (New York: Ballantine Books, 1997), pp. 342–44.

16. Mark Lindley, "Gandhi's Last Words," Bund fuer Geistesfreiheit (Association of Free-Thinkers), http://www.bfg-muenchen.de/rahim.htm (accessed January 24, 2006); and Wahiduddin Richard Shelquist, "Bismillah ir rahman ir rahim," Wahiduddin's Web, October 18, 2005, http://wahiduddin.net/words/bismillah.htm (accessed January 24, 2006).

17. Shizuto Masunaga, *Meridian Exercises*, trans. Stephen Brown (New York: Japan Publications, 1987).

18. Adapted from Christiane Northrup, *Women's Bodies, Women's Wisdom* (New York: Bantam Books, 1994), pp. 80–82; and Anodea Judith and Selene Vega, *The Sevenfold Journey: Reclaiming Mind, Body and Spirit Through the Chakras* (Freedom, CA: The Crossing Press, 1993).

Chapter 6: Vitality

1. Seigen Yamaoka, *The Art and the Way of Hara*, rev. ed. (Union City, CA: Heian International, 1992), pp. 29–30.

2. Stephanie Saul, "Record Sales of Sleeping Pills Are Causing Worries," *New York Times*, February 7, 2006, http://www.nytimes.com/2006/02/07/business/07sleep.html (accessed February 8, 2006).

3. Yamaoka, pp. 30–31.

Chapter 7: Pleasure

1. E. O. Laumann, A. Paik, and R. C. Rosen, "Sexual Dysfunction in the United States: Prevalence and Predictors," *JAMA* 281, no. 6 (February 10, 1999), pp. 537–44.

2. Robert T. Michael, John H. Gagnon, Edward O. Laumann, and Gina Kolata, *Sex in America: A Definitive Survey* (Boston: Little, Brown, 1994), pp. 114–16.

Chapter 9: Compassion

1. Ira Progoff, *At a Journal Workshop* (New York: Dialogue House, 1975).

Chapter 12: Purpose

1. Barbara Ann Brennan, "Our Intentionality and the Hara Dimension," in *Light Emerging: The Journey of Personal Healing* (New York: Bantam, 1993); Irene Claremont de Castillejo, *Knowing Woman: A Feminine Psychology* (Boston: Shambhala, 1997), p. 137; and Tokiko DeSola, personal communication with author, July 1997.

Chapter 14: Restoring Your World

1. *To Wake Up One Day Different: A Conversation Between Ram Das and John Seed*, VHS, directed by Joseph Tieger and Shams Kairys, produced by Rainforest Information Centre (Lismore, Australia: Video Activist Project, 1996).

Appendix 1: Women's Bellies in History and Culture

1. Starhawk, *The Spiral Dance: 20th Anniversary Edition* (San Francisco: Harper and Row, 1999), pp. 30, 232; and Richard J. Green, "How Many Witches?" The Holocaust History Project, December 9, 2000, http://www.holocaust-history.org/~rjg/witches.shtml (accessed January 24, 2006).

2. Barbara Walker, *The Woman's Encyclopedia of Myths and Secrets* (San Francisco: Harper and Row, 1983), p. 1007.

3. U.S. Department of Justice, "Forcible Rape," *Crime in the United States, 2004*, http://www.fbi.gov/ucr/cius_04/offenses_reported/violent_crime/forcible_rape.html (accessed January 24, 2006).

4. International Labour Organization, "Note to Correspondents: International Women's Day," March 5, 2002, http://www.ilo.org/public/english/bureau/inf/pr/2002/8.htm (accessed January 24, 2006).

5. Family Violence Prevention Fund, "The Facts on Reproductive Health and Violence Against Women," p. 1, http://www.endabuse.org/resources/facts/ReproductiveHealth.pdf (accessed January 24, 2006); Centers for Disease Control and Prevention, "Intimate Partner Violence during Pregnancy, A Guide for Clinicians," pp. 2, 12, http://www.cdc.gov/reproductivehealth/violence/IntimatePartnerViolence/ (accessed January 24, 2006); Catherine F. Klein and Leslye E. Orloff, "Providing Legal Protection for Battered Women: An Analysis of State Statutes and Case Law," *Hofstra Law Review* 21 (1993), pp. 801, 827.

6. I. L. Horon and others, "Enhanced Surveillance for Pregnancy-Associated Mortality — Maryland, 1993–1998," *JAMA* 285, no. 11 (March 21, 2001), pp. 1455–59, http://jama.ama-assn.org/cgi/content/abstract/285/11/1455 (accessed January 24, 2006).

7. Centers for Disease Control and Prevention, "Fact Sheet: Hysterectomy in the United States, 1980–1993," August 8, 1997, http://www.cdc.gov/reproductivehealth/WomensRH/FS_Hysterectomy.htm; Centers for Disease

Control and Prevention, "Hysterectomy Surveillance — United States, 1994-1999," July 12, 2002, http://www.cdc.gov/mmwr/preview/mmwrhtml/ss5105a1.htm (accessed January 24, 2006).

8. M. S. Broder and others, "The Appropriateness of Recommendations for Hysterectomy," *Obstetrics & Gynecology* 95, no. 2 (February 2000), pp. 199-205.

9. Centers for Disease Control and Prevention, "Fact Sheet."

10. Ibid.

11. Joyce A. Martin and others, "Births: Final Data for 2003," *National Vital Statistics Reports* 54, no. 2 (Centers for Disease Control and Prevention, September 8, 2005), pp. 15-16, http://www.cdc.gov/nchs/data/nvsr/nvsr54/nvsr54_02.pdf (accessed January 24, 2006); Lauran Neergaard, "Caesareans on the Rise," Associated Press, *The Hannibal Courier-Post*, August 30, 2000, http://www.hannibal.net/stories/083000/new_0830000001.html (accessed January 24, 2006).

12. Rachel Galvin, "Margaret Sanger's 'Deeds of Terrible Virtue,'" Newsletter, National Endowment for the Humanities, September 1998; and Janet Brodie, *Contraception and Abortion in 19th-Century America* (Ithaca, NY: Cornell University Press, 1994).

13. Stanley K. Henshaw, "Unintended Pregnancy in the United States," *Family Planning Perspectives* 30, no. 1 (January/February 1998), pp. 26-27, http://www.agi-usa.org/pubs/journals/3002498.html (accessed January 24, 2006).

14. The Alan Guttmacher Institute, "Get in the Know: Abortion Incidence," September 2005, http://www.guttmacher.org/in-the-know/incidence.html (accessed December 12, 2005).

15. NARAL Pro-Choice America Foundation, "The Safety of Legal Abortion and the Hazards of Illegal Abortion," January 1, 2005, http://www.prochoiceamerica.org/facts/hazards_illegal_abortion.cfm (accessed January 24, 2006).

16. Gena Corea, *The Mother Machine: Reproductive Technologies from Artificial Insemination to Artificial Wombs* (New York: Harper and Row, 1985).

17. Susan M. Duty, Manori J. Silva, Dana B. Barr, John W. Brock, Louise Ryan, Zuying Chen, Robert F. Herrick, David C. Christiani, and Russ Hauser, "Phthalate Exposure and Human Semen Parameters," *Epidemiology* 14, no. 3 (May 2003), pp. 269-77; and Jane A. Hoppin, "Male Reproductive Effects of Phthalates: An Emerging Picture," *Epidemiology* 14, no. 3 (May 2003), pp. 259-60.

18. Samuel Johnson to John Taylor, August 18, 1763, in *Letters of Samuel Johnson*, ed. R. W. Chapman (Oxford: Clarendon Press, 1952), vol. 1, p. 157.

19. Robert Wayne Pelton, *Loony Laws That You Never Knew You Were Breaking* (New York: Walker, 1990), p. 34.

20. The American Society for Aesthetic Plastic Surgery, *2004 Statistics* (New York: Cosmetic Surgery National Data Bank, 2005), pp. 9–13.

21. National Eating Disorders Association, "Statistics: Eating Disorders and Their Precursors" (Seattle: NEDA, 2002), http://www.nationaleating disorders.org/p.asp?WebPage_ID=286&Profile_ID=41138 (accessed January 24, 2006).

22. Ibid.

23. National Center for Health Statistics, "Provisional Data from the Health Promotion and Disease Prevention Supplement to the National Health Interview Survey: United States, January–March 1985," *Vital and Health Statistics*, no. 113 (November 15, 1985), p. 3, http://198.246.96.2/nchs/data/ad/ad113acc.pdf (accessed January 24, 2006).

24. L. M. Mellin and others, "Disordered Eating Characteristics in Preadolescent Girls," paper presented at the annual meeting of the American Dietetic Association, Las Vegas, 1986.

25. National Eating Disorders Association, "Statistics: Eating Disorders and Their Precursors"; and National Association of Anorexia Nervosa and Associated Disorders, "What Causes Eating Disorders?" http://www.anad.org/site/anadweb/content.php?type=1&id=6982 (accessed January 24, 2006).

26. National Eating Disorders Association, "Statistics"; National Organization for Women Foundation Women's Health Project, "Fact Sheet: Women and Eating Disorders," http://loveyourbody.nowfoundation.org/factsheet_2.html (accessed January 24, 2006); Ginia Bellafante, "When Midlife Seems Just an Empty Plate," Fashion and Style, *New York Times*, March 9, 2003, http://www.nytimes.com/2003/03/09/fashion/09EAT.html?pagewanted=1&ei=5070&en=d75741D04302384a&ex=1138424400 (accessed January 24, 2006); and Maryelizabeth Forman, PhD, "A Descriptive Overview of Middle-Aged Women with Eating Disorders," *The Renfrew Perspective*, summer 2004, pp. 1–4.

27. John Barnhill and others, *If You Think You Have an Eating Disorder* (New York: Dell, 1998).

Illustration Sources

All illustrations are by the author. Several of the figures are adaptations of illustrations presented in other works, as referenced below.

Labrys, page 57: Bruce Hartzler, "Labrys," in *Survey of Classical Greek Archaeology*, http://www.hartzler.org/cc307/minoan/images/b4.jpg (accessed January 2, 2006).

Labyrinth, page 57: *Encyclopedia of Religion* (New York: Macmillan, 1987), s.v. "Labyrinth" (by Lima De Freitas), fig. 5.

Tri-line figurine, page 155: Marija Gimbutas, *The Language of the Goddess: Unearthing the Hidden Symbols of Western Civilization* (San Francisco: Harper and Row, 1989), p. 91, fig. 149-2a.

Belly bowl figurine, page 165: Gimbutas, p. 14, fig. 22-1.

Seed-form engraving, page 180: Gimbutas, p. 166, fig. 258-2.

Lily figurine, page 194: Gimbutas, p. 254, fig. 394-2.

Winged figure, page 207: Gimbutas, p. 8, fig. 9-2.

Tree figure, page 219: Gimbutas, p. 17, fig. 28-3.

Ship rock-carving, page 230: Gimbutas, p. 249, fig. 386-7.

Bibliography and Resources

BIBLIOGRAPHY

Baring, Anne, and Jules Cashford. *The Myth of the Goddess*. London: Viking, 1991.

Berg, Miriam. *Facts and Figures*. Mt. Marion, NY: Council on Size and Weight Discrimination, 2003.

Brennan, Barbara Ann. *Light Emerging: The Journey of Personal Healing*. New York: Bantam, 1993.

Camphausen, Rufus C. *The Yoni: Sacred Symbol of Female Creative Power*. Rochester, VT: Inner Traditions, 1996.

Chernin, Kim. *The Obsession: Reflections on the Tyranny of Slenderness*. San Francisco: Harper and Row, 1981.

Claremont de Castillejo, Irene. *Knowing Woman: A Feminine Psychology*. Boston: Shambhala, 1997.

Cohen, Kenneth S. *The Way of Qigong: The Art and Science of Chinese Energy Healing*. New York: Ballantine Books, 1997.

Corea, Gena. *The Mother Machine: Reproductive Technologies from Artificial Insemination to Artificial Wombs*. New York: Harper and Row, 1985.

Dossey, Larry, MD. *Healing Words: The Power of Prayer and the Practice of Medicine*. San Francisco: HarperSanFrancisco, 1993.

Dürckheim, Karlfried Graf von. *Hara: The Vital Centre of Man*. London: Unwin, 1984.

Eisler, Riane. *The Chalice and the Blade: Our History, Our Future.* San
     Francisco: Harper and Row, 1987.
Ellis, Andrew, Niegel Wiseman, and Ken Boss. *Grasping the Wind.* Brookline, MA:
     Paradigm Publications, 1989.
Ensler, Eve. *The Good Body.* New York: Villard/Random House, 2004.
Estés, Clarissa Pinkola. *Women Who Run With the Wolves: Myths and Stories of
     the Wild Woman Archetype.* New York: Ballantine, 1992.
Gadon, Elinor. *The Once and Future Goddess: A Symbol for Our Time.* San
     Francisco: Harper and Row, 1989.
Gershon, Michael D. *The Second Brain.* New York: HarperCollins, 1998.
Gimbutas, Marija. *The Language of the Goddess: Unearthing the Hidden Symbols
     of Western Civilization.* San Francisco: Harper and Row, 1989.
Halifax, Joan. *Shaman Voices: A Survey of Visionary Narratives.* New York: E. P.
     Dutton, 1979.
Hall, Nor. *The Moon and the Virgin: Reflections on the Archetypal Feminine.* New
     York: Harper and Row, 1980.
Hilber, Alison. *Change How You See, Not How You Look.* New Bern, NC:
     Trafford, 2002.
Hollander, Anne. *Seeing Through Clothes.* New York: The Viking Press, 1978.
Judith, Anodea, and Selene Vega. *The Sevenfold Journey: Reclaiming Mind, Body
     and Spirit Through the Chakras.* Freedom, CA: The Crossing Press, 1993.
Kano, Susan. *Making Peace with Food: Freeing Yourself from the Diet/Weight
     Obsession.* New York: Harper Paperbacks, 1989.
Katz, Richard. *Boiling Energy: Community Healing Among the Kalahari Kung.*
     Cambridge, MA: Harvard University Press, 1982.
Kelly, Mary B. *Goddess Embroideries of Eastern Europe.* Winona, MN: Northland
     Press, 1989.
Kilbourne, Jean. *Can't Buy My Love: How Advertising Changes the Way We Think
     and Feel.* New York: Simon and Schuster, 2000.
Lawlor, Robert. *Sacred Geometry: Philosophy and Practice.* London: Thames and
     Hudson, 1982.
———. *Voices of the First Day: Awakening in the Aboriginal Dreamtime.*
     Rochester, VT: Inner Traditions, 1991.
Lubell, Winifred. *The Metamorphosis of Baubo: Myths of Women's Sexual Energy.*
     Nashville, TN: Vanderbilt University Press, 1994.

Masunaga, Shizuto. *Meridian Exercises*. Translated by Stephen Brown. New York: Japan Publications, 1987.

Matsumoto, Kiiko, and Stephen Birch. *Hara Diagnosis: Reflections on the Sea*. Brookline, MA: Paradigm Publications, 1988.

Michael, Robert T., John H. Gagnon, Edward O. Laumann, and Gina Kolata. *Sex in America: A Definitive Survey*. Boston: Little, Brown, 1994.

National Eating Disorders Association, "Statistics: Eating Disorders and Their Precursors," http://www.nationaleatingdisorders.org/p.asp?WebPage_ID=286&Profile_ID=41138 (accessed December 29, 2005).

Noble, Vicki. *Shakti Woman: Feeling Our Fire, Healing Our World — The New Female Shamanism*. San Francisco: HarperCollins, 1991.

Northrup, Christiane. *Women's Bodies, Women's Wisdom*. New York: Bantam Books, 1994.

Oki, Masahiro. *Zen Yoga Therapy*. New York: Japan Publications, 1979.

Post, Allison, and Stephen Cavaliere. *Unwinding the Belly*. Berkeley: North Atlantic Books, 2003.

Progoff, Ira. *At a Journal Workshop*. New York: Dialogue House, 1975.

Rainer, Tristine. *The New Diary*. Los Angeles: J. P. Tarcher, 1978.

Richards, M. C. *Centering: In Pottery, Poetry, and the Person*. Middletown, CT: Wesleyan University Press, 1964.

Starbird, Margaret. *The Woman with the Alabaster Jar: Mary Magdalen and the Holy Grail*. Santa Fe, NM: Bear and Co., 1993.

Starhawk. *The Spiral Dance: 20th Anniversary Edition*. San Francisco: Harper and Row, 1999.

Steele, Valerie. *Fashion and Eroticism: Ideals of Feminine Beauty from the Victorian Era to the Jazz Age*. New York: Oxford University Press, 1985.

Walker, Barbara. *The Woman's Encyclopedia of Myths and Secrets*. San Francisco: Harper and Row, 1983.

———. *The Woman's Dictionary of Symbols and Sacred Objects*. San Francisco: Harper and Row, 1988.

Waters, Frank. *Book of the Hopi*. New York: Penguin Books, 1977.

Wolf, Naomi. *The Beauty Myth: How Images of Beauty Are Used Against Women*. New York: Anchor/Doubleday, 1992.

Yamaoka, Seigen. *The Art and the Way of Hara*, rev. ed. Union City, CA: Heian International, 1992.

RESOURCES

Eating Disorders: Prevention and Treatment

United States: National Eating Disorders Association, 800-931-2237, www.nationaleatingdisorders.org

Canada: National Eating Disorder Information Centre, 866-633-4220 (Toronto: 416-340-4156), www.nedic.ca

Music

Consider these albums and artists when choosing music to accompany your belly-energizing moves:

Earthbeat, Paul Winter Consort, Living Music
Full, Rachel Bagby, Outta the Box
Praises for the World, Jennifer Berezan, Edge of Wonder Records
Returning, Jennifer Berezan, Edge of Wonder Records
Sacred Pleasure, Shawna Carol, Ladyslipper

Video

Belly Buttons: How Are You Still Connected to Your Mother? is available from Judith Selby, PO Box 21, Forest Knolls, CA 94933.

Contact the Author: Keynote Speaking and Other Offerings

Visit www.loveyourbelly.com for information about events, workshops, teacher training, instructional DVDs, other books by the author, and more.

The author also welcomes you to share your "belly stories" and other responses to the material in this book; please understand that she's not able to reply to every message.

Lisa Sarasohn • Self-Health Education
PO Box 1783 • Asheville, NC 28802-1783
www.loveyourbelly.com • lisa@loveyourbelly.com

Index

L

labyrinth, 52, 56–60, *57*
Lamott, Anne, 11
The Language of the Goddess (Gimbutas), 43
laughter
    belly laugh, 87, 162–63
    healing power of, 87, 163
    Let Yourself Laugh (exercise), 163
Lawlor, Robert, 115
laxatives, 74
Letter from the Future (exercise), 256
Let Yourself Laugh (exercise), 163
life force (*qi, prana, spiritus*), 109–18
    belly's sacred power and, 115–17
    hara and, 111, 112, 123
    healing arts and, 110, 112, 118, *119*
    kanda, 112
    kundalini and, 115
    meridians, 112, 118, *119*
    nadis, 112–13, 115
    names for, globally, 110, 115
    power grid for, 112–14
Light Emerging: The Journey of Personal Healing (Brennan), 231
The Lily (newspaper), 161
Lily (exercise), 194–96, *194, 195, 282*
loving your belly, 17–19, 20, 269

M

Making Peace with Food (Kano), xxi
Mary Magdalene, 54, 56
massage: Stay in Touch (exercise), 213
"Matrix Me" (poem) 121–22
Mayer, Emeran, 99–100
Meath, Ireland, stone engraving, *180*
Medicine Eagle, Brooke, 116
meditation
    belly distress, relieving and, 100
    on origins of life, 102–3
menstruation, 49, 80–81, 83
    cramps, breathing to reduce, 96
    ritual and, 80
meridians, 112, 118, *119*
Miller, Elizabeth Smith, 161
mind-body connection, 95–97, 100–101
    chakras and, 118–21, *120*
    meridians and, 118, *119*

mingmen (Life Gate), 105
Moravian winged figure, *207*
mothering and being mothered, 104–6
    relationship with mother, 101

N

naming heroes exercise, 6–7
National Eating Disorders Association (NEDA), 106, 109
National Health and Social Life Survey, 159
Native Americans, 116
nervous system, 88–90
    breathing and, 89
    enteric nervous system (ENS), 90, 97–101
    parasympathetic system, 88, 89
    stress and, 89
    sympathetic system, 88–89
nourishing, 179–83, 263, *180, 182*
    Power Centering, 180–83, *183, 282*

O

Ocean Mother, 102–3
Oki, Masahiro, xix, 128
Oxford English Dictionary, 61

P

Pandora's Box, 62–63
Parks, Rosa, 6
pelvic floor or pelvic diaphragm, 81
    pubococcygeal (PC) muscle, 81–83
Perineal Squeeze, 82–83, 257
perineum, 81, 85–86
peristalsis, 75, 89, 98, 102–3
Persephone, 52–53, 163
Picture Your Heart's Desire (exercise), 33, 225–26
pleasure, xxiv, 34, 121, 127, 129, 159–69
    Belly Bowl (exercise), 167–69, *168, 282*
    Decorate Your Underwear (exercise), 162
    Glowing Globe (exercise), 164
    Let Yourself Laugh (exercise), 163
    Perineal Squeeze (exercise), 82–83, 257
    sex and sexuality, 159–61, 263
    See also holding space
PMS, 96

About the Author

Lisa Sarasohn is a seasoned Kripalu yoga teacher and bodywork therapist. Certified as an instructor in 1979, she served on staff at Kripalu Center for Yoga & Health in Lenox, Massachusetts, from 1981 to 1988. During this time, she shared yoga with thousands of guests, led workshops on a variety of approaches to holistic health, and trained yoga teachers and bodyworkers. Her articles on the body's center, yoga, and health have appeared in such publications as *Yoga Journal*, *SageWoman*, *Radiance*, and *Personal Transformation*. A graduate of Brown University and an award-winning essayist, poet, and public speaker, she has presented workshops on themes expressed in *The Woman's Belly Book* at conferences, colleges, and learning centers, including Omega Institute, Harvard University, the Renfrew Center, and the Sufi School of Healing. She presents keynote speeches and interactive programs for educational organizations, women's centers, and churches. Her website is www.loveyourbelly.com.

NEW WORLD LIBRARY is dedicated to publishing books and other media that inspire and challenge us to improve the quality of our lives and the world.

We are a socially and environmentally aware company, and we make every attempt to embody the ideals presented in our publications. We recognize that we have an ethical responsibility to our customers, our employees, and our planet.

We serve our customers by creating the finest publications possible on personal growth, creativity, spirituality, wellness, and other areas of emerging importance. We serve our employees with generous benefits, significant profit sharing, and constant encouragement to pursue our most expansive dreams. As members of the Green Press Initiative, we print an increasing number of books with soy-based ink on 100 percent postconsumer waste recycled paper. Also, we power our offices with solar energy and contribute to nonprofit organizations working to make the world a better place for us all.

Our products are available
in bookstores everywhere.
For our catalog, please contact:

New World Library
14 Pamaron Way
Novato, California 94949

Phone: 415-884-2100 or 800-972-6657
Catalog requests: Ext. 50
Orders: Ext. 52
Fax: 415-884-2199

Email: escort@newworldlibrary.com
Website: www.newworldlibrary.com